Medicaid EZ

A Guide to Get Those Nursing Home Bills Paid

How Do I Start This?
What Information Do I Need?
What Questions Should I Ask?
How Long Does It Take?

Beverly Huber Albanese
and Heidi L. Macomber

Writers Club Press
San Jose New York Lincoln Shanghai

Medicaid EZ
A Guide to Get Those Nursing Home Bills Paid

Published by Writers Club Press
an imprint of iUniverse.com, Inc.

For information address:
iUniverse.com, Inc.
620 North 48th Street
Suite 201
Lincoln, NE 68504-3467
www.iuniverse.com

Since federal and state laws change frequently, this book was created to provide
accurate information as of the date of publication. This book is sold with the
understanding that the authors are not engaged in rendering legal, accounting,
or other professional service or advice. If legal advice or other expert assistance
is required, the services of a competent professional person should be sought.

ISBN: 0-595-01097-0

Printed in the United States of America

To Frank X. Huber (1921–1994)

Thank you Dad for teaching me the traits that truly matter–honor, integrity, character, courage and perseverance. I know that your guiding hand is still on my shoulder.

Patricia Kneeland Southard (1945-1995)

Thanks to your inspiration. Your thoughts never published.
I dedicate this book to you.

Contents

Acknowledgements ix

Introduction xi

Chapter 1–How Do I Start This? 1

Chapter 2–Starting the Medicaid Process 7

Chapter 3–Medicaid Application 11

Chapter 4–Face-to-Face Interview 17

Chapter 5–Resources/Assets 23

Chapter 6–Income 37

Chapter 7–Ongoing Requirements After A Case Has Been Opened ..45

Appendix A–Medicaid Application Documentation Checklist 51

Appendix B–Recertification/Re-application Checklist 53

Appendix C–Rights and Responsibilities 55

Appendix D–State Agencies on Aging 57

Appendix E–Long Term Care Ombudsmen 71

Appendix F–State Medicaid Offices 85

Glossary 685

Index 693

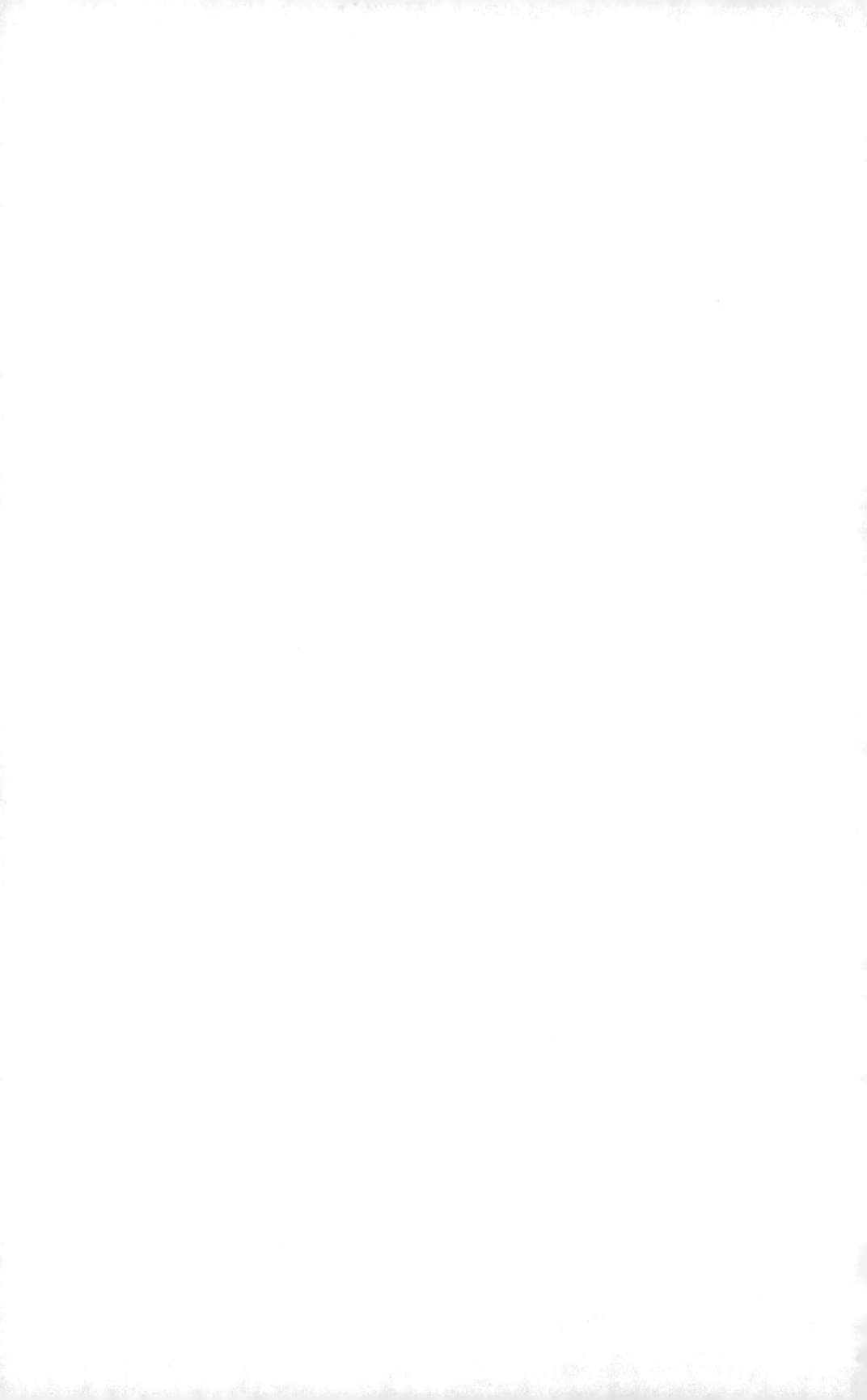

Acknowledgements

THANK YOU GOVERNORS

A big thank you to all of the Governors of the States and also to the Governors of the United States Territories, America Samoa, Guam, Northern Mariana Islands, Puerto Rico, and the Virgin Islands for all of their assistance in providing the requested information regarding their State and Territories. Also to all the people at the various state Medicaid offices that took the time to respond to our technical questions, and the effort to send us the information packets, departmental regulations and administrative code needed to complete this project. Thanks for all the emails, correspondence, and phone calls. We greatly appreciate your help!

Introduction

Growing old is a privilege that most of us will experience. Thanks to science and new health standards, we are living longer these days than ever before. As a result, one of the biggest segments of our population is growing at an ever-increasing rate. The age 65 plus group of people never anticipated that they would live to be a Centurion. Today there are 100,000 people in the United States age 100 and over. The United States Census Bureau estimates this figure to grow to 850,000 by the year 2010. This tremendous growth in the aged portion of the population also means an increase in the number of elderly who will require nursing home care. Most people have no idea that nursing home care can cost as much as $4,000.00 to $7,000.00 a month or more on the average. Medicare for the most part does not pay for nursing home care. The Baby Boomer generation is just starting to get an awareness of what this means as they go through the process of securing nursing home placement for their parents.

Unless you are independently wealthy, you will probably, at some time or another, be faced with applying for Medicaid for nursing home payment. If you know of someone who has applied for Medicaid, you probably have heard that it is a very intimidating and confusing process. You are hit with all of this at the most difficult time, when your parent or family member is very ill. Families are exhausted, confused and feel very vulnerable. There are so many things that need to be done. Coordination of care, changes in daily routine and schedule, and an endless pile of paperwork accompany every decision. One of the biggest

stresses in all of this is dealing with feelings, fears, and personal attach-
ments of the loved one needing the care.

The older generation is very secretive about their finances and feel it
is a real invasion of privacy to disclose all of their private financial
information. Some spouses are left to apply when they have no idea
about the financial piece of their relationship, as the other has always
taken care of things. There is a great sadness when a husband and wife
have been together for most of their lives and now suddenly they are
separated. The thought of having to apply for assistance embarrasses
them as they have always looked after themselves.

This book is a step-by-step guide designed to lead you every step of
the way through the Medicaid process. It speaks specifically to the
patient and their families in understandable terms. The book details
how to begin, who to call, and how to complete the Medicaid application. It provides lists of documentation requirements, checklists,
terms, phone contacts and helpful instructions needed. This is a guide
to prepare you, to help get you organized, and to alleviate some of the
uncertainty and fears you may have in not knowing what to expect. It
is a one-stop source for all that you will need to complete the Medicaid
application process.

Chapter 1
–How Do I Start This?

How-to-Source

Finally, a book that is written for anyone who has questions about applying for Medicaid payment for nursing home or community based waivered services. That would be you, the adult child, spouse, friend of the family, social worker, attorney or advocate. It is a how-to-source for questions and answers about the application process itself, as well as some of the more complicated issues involved with Medicaid eligibility. Most times there are questions about the simplest steps involved. Where do I start? What do I need? How do I do this? Where do I go? Most people do it themselves; others hire attorneys or other specialized representatives. The amount of assets that you own would determine whether you would want to seek the assistance of an attorney or complete the process yourself. We intend to give no legal advice. We do intend to give you the how-to and why for the entire Medicaid process, as well as details and terminology that you should be familiar with.

If you've picked up this book, someone has already told you that it is going to take some work getting the right paperwork together. They were right! Now let's get busy!

What is Medicare, What is Medicaid?

There's a great deal of confusion regarding Medicaid and Medicare. They are not the same programs, and the following will describe each one in detail.

Medicare

Medicare is a federal health insurance program. You apply for this insurance at your local Social Security Office. This program is for the following groups of people. Those who are 65 years old or older, those disabled for at least two years, or have end stage renal disease. If you require an acute level of care, Medicare could possibly pay for a limited amount of days after a three-day hospital stay. It could possibly pay up to 100 days but that decision is based upon the patient's medical condition. Once a patient's level of care has changed from acute care to custodial care, a notice is sent to the patient that on a specified date, Medicare will no longer pay. Please do not be alarmed, as this is a routine practice. Medicare pays based on a person's health condition.

Medicaid

Medicaid is a state and federal health insurance program. You can apply for this program through your local county social services agency. Medicaid will pay for most nursing home costs for people with limited income and resources. Medicaid will only pay for services provided in approved Medicaid nursing home facilities. Medicaid is based on a person's health condition coupled with financial and income guidelines.

What is a Nursing Home?

A nursing home is a facility with the services of professional and qualified technical health personnel such as registered nurses, licensed practical nurses, physical therapists, occupational therapists, speech pathologists, audiologists, etc. A nursing home provides different levels of care for those who have physical and mental impairments, which keep them from living independently.

What are Community Based Waivered Services?

This program is sometimes referred to as the "Nursing Home Without Walls". Health care professionals come into your home to take care of you. This is a program, which provides services to persons at home who would otherwise require institutional care. In order for an individual to be eligible for a home-based waivered service, he/she must require the level of care provided in an institutional setting.

Medical Assessment

You must have a medical necessity as part of the eligibility requirements for Medicaid application. Your doctor determines by your medical condition, whether or not you require long-term placement. A pre-admission screening will be completed to determine the level of care that is appropriate for you. Some of the options could be rehabilitation, home care (commonly referred to as the nursing home without walls), or institutionalized nursing home care. The pre-admission screening is done by various agencies depending on the state where you live. A physician can initiate the pre-admission screening process.

If it has been determined that you require nursing home placement, it is wise to apply to several nursing homes because sometimes there is a wait for an open bed. There are hospital and nursing home staff members who will be very helpful in assisting you. At this time you will be required to complete an application (possibly several) for admittance into the nursing home.

Nursing Home Application Process

When you apply for nursing home care, most times you are already at the hospital and the medical social worker has asked you to list 5 to 7 nursing homes that you might be interested in. You will then have to complete applications for each nursing home. These will require that you list all income and resources. Some of this will be the same information requested on the Medicaid application.

If you are a Medicare/Medicaid recipient applying for admission to a nursing home, it is against the Federal law for a nursing home to require payment of a cash deposit as a condition of admission. After you have applied for Medicaid and are awaiting nursing home placement, you must take the first available nursing home bed. Sometimes it isn't the closest to home or your number one choice, but you can be moved to the nursing home of your choice whenever there is an available bed. The hospital and nursing home staff works very hard to accommodate the patient and their families.

After your application for the nursing home has been received, the hospital/nursing facility, based on the information in your application, will suggest when you need to apply for Medicaid. The hospital that is caring for you at this time will be able to direct you to the local social service office. This is where Medicaid eligibility will be determined. Note; see the state Department of Human Services Medicaid sites under appendices. There is a list of locations where you can apply for Medicaid for each state. Also, for additional information see your state's Office for the Aging and the Ombudsmen program listings. They can provide a variety of services to assist you and your family with the Medicaid application process.

SUMMARY

- What is Medicare, what is Medicaid?
- What is a Nursing Home?
- What are Community Based Waivered Services?
- Medical Assessment
- Nursing Home Application Process

Chapter 2
–Starting the Medicaid Process

Initial Phone Screening-Call Medicaid Representative

Before you make an appointment with the Medicaid department it is usually customary to call and request a phone screening with the Medicaid representative. It is best to be prepared for this phone call by having the information written down and available. You will need to gather together several items. This first call is to determine an estimate of net worth. The Medicaid office will need to know approximately how much the applicant has in combined resources before scheduling an interview. The Medicaid representative will determine by the phone screening an approximate time to apply for Medicaid. At the time when you place the call to the Medicaid department for an interview, you will be asked several questions.

*   *   *

List of information you will need when you call the Medicaid department:

- Patient name
- Marital status
- Has there been a medical determination that the patient is appropriate for nursing home placement?

- Name of hospital/nursing home
- Address where living prior to being admitted into a facility
- Is Medicare or private insurance paying for nursing home care at this time?
- Current balances in savings, checking, investment accounts, stocks, bonds, etc.
- Real estate
- Has there been any cash, income, real estate, or personal property given away in the past 36 months or has a trust been created in the past 60 months, commonly referred to as transfer of resources?

*   *   *

The Medicaid representative will determine by the information given if it is an appropriate time to make an appointment for a face-to-face interview. If the Medicaid representative determines that the time is appropriate, the appointment is scheduled. You will be sent an application, informational notices and instructions as to what information to bring with you to the interview.

What if my resources are more than the state allowance at the time of the phone screening?

The Medicaid representative will need to know how much you have in outstanding medical bills. Usually the biggest one is the nursing home bill. Medicaid compares your total resources to the state allowance and then subtracts the outstanding medical bills. You might have too much in resources. There may be a mutual understanding between the applicant and the Medicaid representative that it is too soon to apply. At this point the application for Medicaid could be premature.

What if I don't have a medical bill yet, but the nursing home keeps asking me if I've applied for Medicaid?

The Medicaid representative may tell you that it is too soon to apply if you have stated that Medicare and other private insurance are currently paying for the medical expenses. The representative will ask if you have received a notice from Medicare that the payment for your care will cease. This is commonly referred to as the Medicare cut letter. Don't be alarmed when you receive this notice, as this is a routine procedure.

Too soon?

Even though it has been determined that it is too soon to apply, it is not too soon to start gathering all of the paperwork that is required to complete the Medicaid application process. It is a legal requirement that the Medicaid representative receive the financial records in order to determine eligibility. This will be a good time to gather all documents to find out what you have and what is still missing. If there are any bank account statements or financial records missing, you will have to request them from the bank. This can sometimes take several weeks, especially if you need records from an out of state bank. The banks may charge you a fee to print duplicate bank statements or records.

Any time you can save will be very worthwhile and to your benefit. The clock starts ticking from the date of the first face-to-face appointment. You will be given a certain amount of time to get all missing items to the Medicaid representative. It can be approximately 20 to 45 days depending on the state where you reside. If you fail to do so, you may receive a denial for failure to provide information requested. This could mean you would have to go through the entire Medicaid application process all over again.

SUMMARY

- Initial phone screening-call Medicaid Representative
- List of questions associated with the phone screening
- Get prepared now

Chapter 3
–Medicaid Application

State Residency Requirements

You must be a resident of a particular state to apply for Medicaid in that state. As a factor of eligibility, an individual who is applying for Medicaid must be living in the state voluntarily and intending to make that particular state his/her home.

In the process of comparing the information on applications from each state, we have compiled a general list of common questions that you will find on the application. Some states have a generic application form, which means everyone uses the same form when applying for public assistance, food stamps, and/or Medicaid. If your state has a generic application form it would be wise for you to call your Medicaid representative and ask if you are required to complete all of the sections of the application (as some may be non-applicable to your situation). State that you are specifically applying for nursing home or community based waivered services. Complete the application form in ink. Answer the questions but do not write in the shaded areas.

*   *   *

The following is a list of commonly asked questions found on a Medicaid application and instructions to assist you in completing the form.

- What is the applicant's name, address, county, state, zip code, and phone number.
- Name, birth date, sex, race, social security number, for yourself, your spouse if you are married, and any dependent children or siblings. You must complete this information for anyone who is applying.
- How long have you been at this address?
- What is/was your previous address?
- There will be a section of questions pertaining to your US Citizen status. If you are not a citizen you will need additional information relating to your alien status.
- Veteran status-are you a veteran or the spouse of a veteran, name the branch of service, date entered, discharge date.
- Income section-there will be a list of income sources that you will need to check a yes or no to. If you check yes to the question, you will need to fill in the amount of the income received per month from the source checked. This section also asks for your spouse and dependent's income as well. Usually they are looking for monthly figures. If you never receive a statement, look for an address and benefit number on previous correspondence. You may need to call or write to request proof of the gross monthly amount.
- Asset/resource section-complete the resource section by answering all of the questions. If for example, you have a savings account you will need to list the current balance, whose name is on the account, and the name of the bank. This holds true of all assets that you own yourself or jointly with others. Some applications also have a spot to list all accounts that have closed out in the past 36 months. Make a note to yourself here to find out where money from these accounts was spent. Medicaid will ask you.

- Has anyone (including your spouse even if not applying or living with you) given away any cash, or sold/transferred any real estate, income or personal property in the past 36 months? Or, has anyone created a trust in the past 60 months? If yes, when? Explain circumstances. It is a good idea to write this explanation down on a separate piece of paper and attach any proof you might have.
- Do you have any unpaid medical bills for the three months preceeding the month of application? They are looking for medical bills with a date of service that falls within the 3-month period prior to the month you are applying for assistance.
- Do you have Medicare and/or secondary health insurance? If so, provide the insurance subscriber number, which appears on your insurance card and the cost of the insurance per month. Do you have long term care insurance? Bring the insurance cards and a recent bill.
- Have you applied for assistance in the past? Have you ever applied for cash, medical or food stamp benefits in another county in the state? You may already have a Medicaid Identification Number and possible information already on file that can help the Medicaid representative.

*   *   *

Please read the back of the application form carefully. This is where you will find a list of your rights, responsibilities, certifications, and consent. There are many variations on the back of the application form depending on the state. The patient may sign the back of the application form, but if unable, a family member or other representative may sign on their behalf. Please find below a breakdown of the information provided on the back of the application form.

Statements of responsibility on the back of the application form:

- You must provide a social security number for all persons included on the application. If you do not have a social security number, you must apply for one. It is usually a good idea to provide proof from the Social Security Administration that you've done so. Your social security number will be used to obtain information to verify your income and resources, etc. You are giving your consent to the department of social services to investigate any information that you have given to them.
- You agree to file any claims for health or accident insurance benefits for which you are entitled to. You also agree to turn over to the state any health insurance payments that you receive while on Medicaid. You are authorizing Medicare Part B payments to go directly to doctors and medical providers. Medicaid does not pay medical expenses that your private health insurance company is responsible to pay.
- You may be required to repay the cost of medical assistance services received (to pay for nursing facility services, home and community-based waivered services and any related hospital and prescription drug services) from your probate estate.
- You need to report to the agency any changes in income, any lump sum or windfall income, increases in your health insurance premium, changes in your marital status, changes of address, etc. These changes must be reported as soon as possible.
- Please answer all questions truthfully. Provide information that is true, correct and complete. There are penalties involved if you give fraudulent information.

*　　　　　*　　　　　*

Again, please read the back of the Medicaid application form carefully. The above lists the major points of information. You will be signing the application form verifying that you have read and understand the information that is listed on the back of the form. Your Medicaid representative should review the application form with you at the interview and answer any questions you may have.

SUMMARY

- State residency requirements
- How to complete the application
- Details on how to complete the income and resource sections
- Health insurance information
- Break down of points of information which appear on the back of the Medicaid application
- Information supporting the fact that you've read and understand the back of the Medicaid application form, which requires a signature

Chapter 4
–Face-to-Face Interview

What is a face-to-face interview?

If you have determined that your state requires a face-to-face interview (by your call to the social service agency), you will need to set up a time for your Medicaid eligibility interview. You should plan on a few hours for the interview. You will need to bring with you the completed and signed application along with the required documentation. Note; do not reschedule the appointment if you are missing documentation. The Medicaid representative is required to give you time to provide the missing information.

Who must attend the interview?

A family member or friend of the patient may do the interview on behalf of the patient. The patient is not expected to appear at the interview. Please be on time for your appointment. When you arrive for your appointment give your name to the receptionist. Since the social services offices are very busy, after waiting approximately 15 minutes without being called, it is a good idea to remind the receptionist about your scheduled appointment.

The Interview

Once the interview has started, the Medicaid representative will ask you questions pertaining to the completed application. Actually, you will be asked the same questions that you were asked on the application, but you will then be expected to verify the information with the documentation that you gathered and brought with you. The Medicaid representative will explain the program, income, resources, transfers, penalties, the back of the form, and any questions that you may have. You will be given several handouts. You will probably feel overwhelmed by all of the information. When you return home and think of questions that you didn't ask, you can always call for clarification. Your Medicaid representative is there to help you. If you are missing required documentation at the time of the interview you will be given additional time. Please be advised that it is very important that you send in the additional information within this time frame. Failure to do so could result in a denial of your Medicaid application.

*   *   *

List of documentation to bring with you to your face-to-face interview:

- Records showing age-birth certificate, baptismal record, census record.
- Record of place of birth, or if foreign born, record of naturalization or Alien status.
- If married-copy of marriage certificate.
- If divorced-copy of divorce decree.
- If widow/widower-copy of death certificate, obituary notice, or mass card.
- Copy of social security card.

- Copy of Medicare card and health insurance card. Also, if you are paying for your secondary health insurance, you will need current verification of the amount that you pay.
- Copy of power of attorney paperwork (if there is a power of attorney appointed).
- Copy of guardianship papers (if there is a guardian appointed).
- Verification of social security income such as a copy of the social security check; if direct deposited in bank account, a copy of the bank statement; or a copy of the award letter from social security.
- Wage income-you will need copies of check stubs, which show gross and net income. You will probably have to provide at least 4 consecutive weeks of salary information.
- Retirement pensions–copy of check stub showing gross and net retirement income or letter from your pension company verifying your pension income.
- Dividends, interest-income tax returns, 1099's, or letters from the various financial institutions with the stated income.
- You will need to provide records for any other income, which you receive from any other source.
- You will need to provide 36 months of bank records for all open and closed accounts; records of stocks, bonds, and other assets for the 36 months prior to the month coverage is needed.
- You will need to provide 60 months of financial records for trusts and annuities.
- You will need to provide copies of life insurance policies and current cash values of those policies. Contact your local life insurance representative to request verification.
- You will need to provide records for burial funds and burial spaces. Funeral director can help you.
- If you own real estate, you will need to provide copies of deeds, and current tax information. You will need to provide shelter expenses if your state has a shelter allowance. If you have sold real estate

within the 36-month look-back period you will need a copy of the closing statement for the sale of the property. You will also need proof of the fair market value (an appraisal) at the time of the sale.

- Copies of titles or registrations for vehicles and recreational vehicles.
- A statement of contents if you have a safe deposit box (usually a notarized statement).
- You must provide documentation of your residence prior to going to a nursing home. Look for address verification on current mail, i.e. bank statements, or possible receipts for rent and/or taxes for home ownership.
- Copies of medical bills for the three months prior to the application.

*   *   *

If you are having problems getting together the required documentation, your Medicaid representative could be of some help. Another source to help you would be your local Office for the Aging. In the appendix section of this book there is a list of all the State Agencies on Aging. By calling your state Office for the Aging you will be given the number for your local agency. Usually hospitals and nursing home facilities have staff members who will be able to assist you. Please remember that there is no wiggle room in providing income and financial records. You must furnish all financial records requested. We recommend getting help from as many sources as you can.

You've done your part

You've done your part and now it's up to the Medicaid representative to do theirs. This process can take approximately 30 to 45 days to complete. The applicant/patient representative will be notified by mail when the process has been completed. If you have been approved, you will be sent a "Notice of Eligibility" letter from the agency. This notice will give you the effective date and the amount of patient contribution towards costs of care. The medical facility will also get a copy of this letter of eligibility. They will send a new bill according to the opening notice. All payments owed will go to the nursing home, not the Medicaid office. Maintenance of checking account, savings, etc. can continue without change. Speak with the social worker at the nursing home if you no longer wish to handle these transactions. Sometimes arrangements can be made by the social worker for the nursing home to become representative payee and take over all or some of the financial accountability for you. The income can be sent directly to the nursing home. They will take out the personal needs amount and health insurance premium and apply the remainder of the income to the cost of care per month.

Fair hearing

If you have been denied and you disagree with this determination, you have a right to request a fair hearing. A fair hearing is a meeting that is usually held at the local social service agency. The persons attending the fair hearing are the applicant's representative, the Medicaid representative, and the Fair Hearing Officer. The Medicaid representative will state the agency's position, and the representative of the applicant will be able to state their rebuttal. The fair hearing officer will make a determination and the agency and the applicant will be notified of the decision. The instructions for the procedures to request a fair hearing should be listed on your notice from the agency. It is important to pay attention to the time frame required for the request as it could expire. As a result of failing to adhere to the time element given, it could mean that you will have to re-apply for Medicaid payment.

Summary

- What is a face-to-face interview?
- Who must attend the interview?
- The Interview
- List of required documentation
- You've done your part
- Right to a fair hearing

Chapter 5
–Resources/Assets

Resource/assets

A "resource" is defined as cash or liquid assets and real or personal property. A liquid resource is an asset, which can readily be converted to cash. A non-liquid resource is an asset or property, which cannot readily be converted to cash.

There will be a Medicaid resource dollar amount limit, depending upon your marital status, and the state in which you live. If you are married there is a spousal impoverishment law to protect the spouse living at home from being impoverished by medical expenses incurred by the spouse in the nursing home. This law protects a portion of the income and resources for the spouse living at home. Some states have minimum and maximum levels of non-exempt asset limits. This means that they consider the combined resources owned by both the spouses. The stay at home spouse gets one-half of the assets with a minimum of $16,824.00 (2000 level subject to change). If they own less than $16,824.00 the community spouse would get all of the assets. If they own more, the maximum level that the community spouse is entitled to is $84,120.00 (2000 level subject to change). If they own more than $84,120.00, the remaining amount of combined resources is considered available to the institutionalized spouse. There is a set amount that the institutionalized spouse may retain. Your local Medicaid representative would have that amount available as per the state in which you reside.

The remainder over the level would be applied to the institutionalized spouse's cost of care, meaning they would have to spend down the excess (or remainder) on nursing home care before Medicaid would pay.

There are other states that have an $84,120.00 maximum resource level without a minimum level. For example, the community spouse could be entitled to $84,120.00, the homestead, one automobile, a burial account, and $1,500.00 face value life insurance. The resources are not divided in half. The amount over the $84,120.00 would be applied to the institutionalized spouse's asset level. Again, your Medicaid representative would be able to give you those levels based on the state in which you reside.

First of the Month Rule

Countable resources are determined as of the first moment of the month. Note, they really do mean the first moment. The determination is based on the resources the individuals own, their value, and whether or not they are excluded as of the first moment of the month. The first of the month rule establishes a point of time at which to value resources. The value of resources can change during a month but the change is always effective with the following month's resource determination. An example of this is the value of a stock can increase or decrease within the month, or a person can close a bank account within the month. An individual might replace an exempt resource with one that is not exempt, such as selling an automobile for cash.

The snapshot

Snapshot of resources for spousal cases is a term used by Medicaid when determining total assets owned at the time of institutionalization or the date on the Medicaid application, whichever comes first. All assets are considered. After eligibility has been determined and the case is opened, the community spouse's resources are not looked at again except to verify his/her income. If the community spouse decides to give his assets away he/she runs the risk of requiring nursing home care himself within the 36-month look-back period of his/her own application for Medicaid. This is a risk that should be thought about carefully. For any legal advice contact an elder law attorney. The community spouse will be asked to verify income received from his/her assets on an ongoing basis as long as the Medicaid case remains open. For example, if after the Medicaid case is opened and the community spouse wins the lotto, the Medicaid case would not close unless the income generated from the winnings exceeded the allowable Medicaid standards. Remember, you are expected to report to the agency any increase in earnings.

Higher resource level for community spouse

In some circumstances, if the community spouse has the maximum resource level but is below the income level, the community spouse may be able to retain a higher resource level to generate more interest income. A fair hearing or court order must determine this increased resource level. This decision is not made at the local Medicaid level. However, that is where you would make the request.

Married couple residing in a nursing home

If a husband and wife are both residing in a nursing home, the resources are usually treated as if they were both of a single status. Some state levels allow, for example $2,000.00 for each and other states allow a combined $3,000.00 for the couple. The amount varies from state to state.

*   *   *

Examples of resources/assets

- Annuities
- Automobiles, recreational vehicles, trucks, and motorcycles
- Bank accounts
- Burial accounts, burial space
- Cookie jar funds, etc.
- Escrow accounts at nursing home
- Ira's, Keoghs, 401K's
- Life insurance
- Mutual funds
- Real estate
- Savings bonds
- Stocks and bonds
- Trusts

*   *   *

There can be additional unique resources considered depending on the particular state. For example other resources might include oil royalties or mineral rights, livestock, farm machinery, etc.

Look-Back Period

You will need to provide financial records for all resources during what is called the "look back period". The look back period for financial records for all open and closed accounts is 36 months from the date nursing home coverage or community waivered services is needed. You will be asked to submit 60 months of financial records for a Trust.

The following is a list of the most common resources and how these resources will be treated with regard to the Medicaid process.

Annuities

An annuity is usually treated as a trust. For Medicaid purposes; that is, it will be looked at as both an income and a resource. The Medicaid representative will ask for 60 months worth of financial records, and the original contract. It will be important to provide this, as the agency will need to calculate whether or not the initial setting up of the annuity should be considered as a transfer of resources. For example, the monthly payment criteria multiplied by the months already received will tell the Medicaid representative how much you have already received from the arrangement. If you have received more than the original or principal amount invested, then there will be no penalty. If you have received less, then the representative will need to calculate a possible penalty based upon a life expectancy chart. It would be possible to set-up an annuity for a minimum payment option where you would die far before the principal had ever been used up. In this case the agency would calculate how much you gave up or intended for a beneficiary, and use this figure to calculate a penalty. You will have to prove whether or not the annuity is revocable. Check with your Medicaid representative. This has nothing to do with the penalty, just the issues of being over the resource limit because all assets in a revocable annuity will be counted towards the resource limit.

Automobiles, recreational vehicles, trucks and motorcycles

One automobile is excluded as a resource when the individual or member of his/her family uses it. If the automobile is not being used, there is a $4,500.00 deduction from the value, and the remainder is considered a resource. If you feel that the book value is more than the actual trade-in value of the vehicle, you may obtain an appraisal from a reputable dealer. Check with the Medicaid representative for more details.

Bank accounts

Checking, savings, NOW accounts, individual retirement account (IRAs), Keogh and 401K accounts, certificates of deposit, money market accounts, Christmas club, vacation club, stocks, bonds, and mutual funds are tangible accounts which can be readily converted to cash. The balances of these accounts will be considered as part of the total resource level.

Burial accounts

There are many different rules for establishing a burial account depending on which state you live in. Some states have a limit as to how much you are entitled to deposit in a burial account. There are two common types of burial accounts, revocable and irrevocable. Irrevocable basically means that you cannot cancel the account and withdraw the funds. In some states you are limited to $1,500.00 dollars in a revocable account, and anywhere from $1,500.00 to $5,400.00 and up in an irrevocable account. There are some states that have no limit to the amount that is deposited in an irrevocable burial account.

Escrow accounts at nursing homes

Escrow accounts are cash deposits made at the nursing home, prior to admission, if on a self-pay status. Once application for Medicaid has been made this escrow account is considered as a resource and counts against the total resource level.

Household goods and personal effects

Furniture, major appliances, television sets, jewelry, furs, musical instruments, etc. Some states count these items as resources and other states consider these items as exempt. We have found that in some states household and personal items are treated differently from county to county within the state. The applications usually ask for specifics and an estimate of value. Most of the time this is not an issue unless there are valuable antiques and collectibles involved. This is one of those questions to ask for details about in the initial phone screening.

Inheritances, settlements, lump sums, windfalls

If the nursing home patient should receive an inheritance, settlement, lump sum or windfall, verification of the amount received should be sent to the Medicaid represent immediately. Verification of the amount received would depend on the type of award received. A copy of the letter (sent from an attorney), that usually accompanies the check, would be appropriate. Generally, the lump sum payments are considered as income in the month received and then counted as a resource in any subsequent month. It would be wise to check with your Medicaid representative for clarification immediately upon notification of the award.

Life insurance

Generally, you are entitled to $1,500.00 face value life insurance that will not be counted towards your resources. If you have several life insurance policies and the total of the face values are at or below $1,500.00 those policies will not be counted towards your resource limit. The cash value is considered if the face value of the insurance policies exceeds $1,500.00. The amount over the $1,500.00 would be considered a countable resource. Sometimes your life insurance is tied in with your burial account depending on which state you live in. Term insurance and group insurance have no cash value provisions and are, therefore, not counted as a resource.

Real estate

A homestead is the principal place of residence. The homestead is not counted during periods when the institutionalized individual is in an acute care or long-term care medical facility and intends to return home. If the institutionalized individual is not able to return home the homestead is exempt if there is a spouse or a dependent relative living in the home. If the institutional individual has no intent to return home and there is no spouse or dependent relative living in the home, the home is considered a countable asset. The home must be sold at fair market value. The proceeds from the sale of the home (after the institutionalized individual's bank account has been brought up to the appropriate resource level and arrangements have been made to establish a burial account) must be applied to the individual's cost of care. Check with your local Medicaid representative and she/he will direct you with the best approach to take. If you have other property such as a second home or cottage for your recreational use, this would be counted as an asset.

Trusts

If you have created a trust in the past 60 months, be prepared to provide the following documentation at the time of your Medicaid eligibility interview:

*   *   *

- Sixty months of financial records relating to the trust.
- Copies of the entire trust agreement with all amendments and statements.
- Inventories of trust assets.
- A Schedule A or other trust documentation listing the income or resources assigned to the trust at the time that the trust was created.

- Date the trust was funded.
- A list of the name and address of all trustees.
- Verification of whether income and resources assigned to the trust have been legally titled to the trust.
- Verification of current cash value of all resources assigned and titled to the trust.
- Verification of current income assigned to the trust and trust disbursements.
- There could be additional information specifically requested by your local agency.

*　　　　*　　　　*

This documentation is required so that the Medicaid agency can make a determination if this trust is within the guidelines of the Medicaid regulations. Based on the type of trust you have created and the date that the trust was funded, there is a possibility that a penalty period could be imposed. The Medicaid representative is going to determine the income that you receive from the trust and if any part of the trust can be counted as a resource.

6% rate of return

The 6% rate of return test can reduce a certain amount of the equity value of income producing property. Note that this may help to reduce the countable value of a property asset; it is not a means of reducing the income generated from the property. For example, if the annual net income is at least 6% of the equity value of the property, the first $12,000 of equity value is not a countable resource. If annual net income is less than 6% of the equity value, the entire equity value is a countable resource. See the following example:

*　　　　*　　　　*

Rental Property	Fair market Value	$51,000
	Outstanding Mortgage	-35,000
	Equity Value	$16,000
		X 0.06
		$ 960
Net annual income from rental property		$1,000

*   *   *

Because net annual income ($1,000.00) is more than 6% of the equity value of the rental property ($960.00), $12,000.00 of the equity value is exempted leaving $4,000.00 as a countable resource. If this is something that might apply to your situation, please check with your Medicaid representative for specific details in your State.

Transfer of resources (if you have given away cash, real estate or personal property in the past 36 months).

If you or your spouse has given away cash, real estate or personal property or sold an asset for less than fair market value in the past 36 months prior to applying for Medicaid you could face a penalty period. During the penalty period Medicaid would not pay for the nursing home bed. The penalty period is determined by dividing the amount of the transfer by the average going nursing home rate (in the area).

*   *   *

Example:
A $24,000.00 transferred amount divided by $3,000.00 going nursing home rate equals eight months of a penalty period from the date of the transfer. Some states start counting the penalty period on the first of the month after the date of the transfer. During this time of penalty, Medicaid would not pay for the nursing home bed. If this is the case, be sure to ask if you would qualify for medical assistance that

would cover ancillary charges (medical bills for other care and services that are not included in the nursing home's per diem rate). If your state has this policy they will be looking at your total resources and net income to determine eligibility.

*   *   *

There are acceptable transfers such as:
- The transfer of a home or other assets from spouse to spouse.
- The transfer of assets to a blind or disabled son or daughter.
- The transfer of a home to a son or daughter under 21 years of age.
- The transfer of a home to a brother or sister who has an equity interest in the home and who has lived in the home for at least one year immediately prior to your entering the nursing home.
- The transfer of a home to a son or daughter, who has lived in the home and has provided care for the parent, which has delayed the need for nursing home care for at least two years.
- Creating a trust for the sole benefit of a blind or disabled person under age 65.

What if?

Here is another acceptable transfer. At the time of the transfer the applicant had no expectation of applying for Medicaid and the resources were transferred exclusively for a purpose other than to qualify for Medicaid.

*   *   *

Example:

If your mother gave you $40,000.00 in January while she was in good health and of sound mind, and had a stroke in March of the same year, and ended up in a nursing home, there would be no penalty. The reason being is she had no idea at the time of the gift that she would suddenly become ill and need nursing home coverage. Medicaid may not consider this a pre-meditated transfer of assets. She did not try to get rid of assets in order to qualify for Medicaid. To verify this, you need supporting documentation (such as a statement from your mother's doctor) that at the time of the gift she was in good health and of sound mind.

The Medicaid representative will review the documentation and make a decision. If the decision is not in your favor, you will be given an opportunity to rebut the agency's presumption that the transfer was done for the sole purpose of becoming eligible for Medicaid. If after the Medicaid representative reviews your letter of rebuttal and believes that it was a premeditated transfer to qualify for Medicaid, you have the right to request a fair hearing.

If an asset is given away without a fair market return and the applicant is placed on restricted Medicaid coverage, there are options to re-establish full Medicaid coverage. The person who received the resource can reimburse the applicant for the asset at fair market value. Also, the asset can be transferred back to the applicant. The asset can be sold at fair market value by the individual to whom the asset was transferred, with the proceeds applied to the applicant's cost of care.

Life estate

If you transferred your home prior to the 36 month look back period but have retained life use, you are entitled to a portion of the proceeds if the house is sold based on the "unisex life estate and remainder interest tables". If the house is rented you are entitled to the net rental income, which will be applied to your cost of care.

SUMMARY

- Explanation of the terms Resource/Assets
- First of the Month Rule
- The Snapshot
- Higher Resource Level
- Married Couple residing in a Nursing Home
- Look Back Period
- Examples of Resources
- 6% Rate of Return Test
- Transfer of Resources (giving away cash, real estate or personal property)
- Life Estate

Chapter 6
-Income

Single, divorced, widow/widower treatment of income

If you are single, divorced, widow/widower, your income will be applied to the monthly cost of your nursing home care. You are entitled to various deductions from your income. Each state has a deduction commonly called a personal needs deduction. For example your state might have a personal needs deduction in the amount of $50.00. This $50.00 per month is your spending money (there are different amounts depending on the state). Maybe you would want to use it to get your hair done, buy personal items, and pay for telephone calls and cable TV, etc. This personal need amount is yours to use for whatever you want. There is also a deduction from your income for your medical insurance premiums. Medicaid would like you to keep your secondary medical insurance in place so this deduction would allow you enough money each month to pay your premiums. You are also entitled to a deduction from your income if you have a dependent (child, sibling, etc.).

*　　　　　*　　　　　*

Example of monthly contribution to the nursing home for cost of care:

$745.50	gross social security amount
-45.50	Medicare
-70.00	health insurance premium per month
$630.00	
-50.00	personal needs allowance
$580.00	amount you will pay the nursing home per month for cost of care

Additional deductions from income depending on the state where you reside.

- If you own your own home and your intent is to return there, some states have a home maintenance allowance that can be deducted from your income to help you with your expenses relating to your home.
- If there has been a guardian appointed by the courts on your behalf, you are entitled to a deduction for guardian fees. Your local Medicaid representative will be able to assist you with questions regarding other deductions from your income.

Miller trusts, or income trusts

There are certain "income cap" states that allow Miller trusts or income trusts as a means of qualifying for Medicaid when one would otherwise be over the allowable monthly income limit. This applies to states that would normally deny an applicant who has as little as $1.00 over the income limit. Only income can be placed in the trust. The trust must be irrevocable. Distributions can then be made towards a person's cost of care (or contribution for Medicaid purposes). Any funds left in the trust at death go to repay Medicaid. An attorney is required to establish a Miller Trust.

Income guidelines for married couples

If both a husband and wife are placed in a nursing home, their income is treated as if they are both single. Each would pay a certain cost of care to the nursing home monthly with the applicable deductions as listed above. If one spouse is home and the other is in the nursing home or receiving home care, the income is treated differently.

A community spouse is entitled to a certain amount of income per month based on the income level set forth by the state in which they reside. An institutionalized person who applies for Medicaid is entitled to protect some of their income by transferring it to the community spouse. You can transfer only if the community spouse is below the established income level. New York State, for example, has a $2,103.00 per month income level for the community spouse (2000). If after the medical insurance premiums and the personal need allowances are deducted, the net income is below the $2,103.00, the institutionalized spouse's income may be transferred to the community spouse. You can only transfer enough to bring him/her up to the level or closer to the level of $2,103.00. This may result in no cost of care payment to the nursing home per month. However, if the community spouse's income were at $2,103.00 per month, the institutionalized spouse's income minus the standard deductions (listed above) would be paid to the nursing home towards cost of care monthly.

In some states there is a standard level of income for the community spouse or a lower level coupled with an "excess shelter allowance". The excess shelter allowances change each year. The excess shelter allowance includes expenses for rent, mortgage principal and interest, and taxes and insurance for your place of residency. If the community spouse lives in a condominium, there could be an allowance for the monthly maintenance charges and utilities paid by the community spouse. Any income above the level (after the specified deductions are considered) would go to the nursing home as a monthly cost of care payment.

In some states the community spouse's monthly income is not counted. This income could be above the established level. If the community spouse's income is below the state's established income level it would be counted to determine how much of the institutionalized spouse's income would need to be attributed to bring the community spouses income up to the established level.

What is considered income?

- Alimony
- Annuities
- Black lung
- Cash contributions
- Child support
- German/Austrian reparation payments
- Income from loans
- Interest/dividend income
- IRA's, Keoghs, 401K's
- Lump sum payments
- Oil/gas mineral royalties
- Railroad retirement
- Rental income
- Retirement pensions
- Social security
- Trust income
- Unemployment compensations
- Veteran's pension
- Wages
- Workers' compensation
- Other, etc.

*   *   *

Documentation, which will verify income

- Social security checks-copy of check or copy of yearly award letter.
- Pension checks-check stub or letter describing gross and net benefit.
- Interest income/dividends-copies of 1099's, statements from financial institutions, income tax returns.

- Wages-last 4 week consecutive wage check stubs.
- Rental income-verification of rent received such as a copy of lease agreement, letter from tenant describing amount of rent paid per month. Verification of mortgage payments, taxes, insurance, copies of bills for repairs, maintenance expenses, etc.
- Mortgage income-copy of amortization schedule.
- Workers' compensation/disability payments-copies of award letters.
- Alimony/child support-copies of letters from the courts describing income.
- Self-employed income-copies of income tax statement, copies of business ledgers describing income and expenses.
- Other income-please ask your Medicaid representative what is appropriate to verify the income.

Rental property income

Rental income will be considered as part of your monthly income. To verify the monthly rental income you will probably be asked to provide a copy of a lease agreement. If there is no lease agreement in place you will be asked for a statement from the renter verifying the amount paid to you for the monthly rent. It is always helpful to provide the agency with a copy of your current tax return. You will be entitled to various deductions to arrive at the net monthly rental amount. Ordinary and necessary expenses may include mortgage, taxes, insurance payments, maintenance and repairs, management fees, legal expenses, etc. You will be required to submit documentation to support these expenses. If you have a question pertaining to a certain expense that you're not sure of please contact your local Medicaid representative.

Self-employment/business income

Like any other type of income, you will be required to verify to the agency your self-employment/business income. Types of verification include income tax returns, accountant statements, business records or ledgers, or signed financial statements. If you have a formal partnership agreement you will need to provide the terms and conditions of the agreement. For specifics relating to self-employment/business income guidelines in your state, please check with your local Medicaid representative for clarification.

Veteran's benefits

Veterans and their spouses should contact their local veteran's administration to inquire about the possibility that they could qualify for a veteran's benefit. A married veteran may be entitled to a pension if within a certain income range. If you are a veteran or a widow/widower of a veteran and in a nursing home, you may qualify for a $90.00 a month (aid and attendance) stipend. This $90.00 a month is considered spending money for you to use in addition to your personal needs allowance from your income. This $90.00 a month is exempt from the amount that you owe to the nursing home each month for your cost of care.

Report all changes to income and health insurance premiums as soon as possible

Remember to report all changes of your income such as cost-of-living increases, increases in your pensions, dividends, new sources of income, cash gifts, inheritances, etc. If your health insurance premium should increase you need to report this to your Medicaid representative. The changes need to be reported as soon as possible so that your monthly cost share to the nursing home will be correct. Your Medicaid representative will determine your cost share and send a letter to you and to the nursing home with the new amount based on the change.

If you are entitled to certain income-you must apply for that income

Medicaid Regulations state that you must apply for any income that you might be entitled to. This includes, but is not limited to, retirement pensions, social security, rental income, mortgage income, workers' compensation, disability payments, veteran's benefits, alimony, child support, income from life insurance, etc.

Medicaid applicants who are eligible for periodic retirement benefits must apply for such benefits as a condition of eligibility. If there are a variety of payment options, the individual must choose the maximum income payment that could be made available over the individual's lifetime. By federal law, if the Medicaid applicant has a spouse, the maximum income payment option for a married individual will usually be less than the maximum income payment option that is available to a single individual. A retirement fund owned by an individual is a countable resource if the individual is not entitled to periodic payments, but is allowed to withdraw any of the funds.

Summary

- Single, divorced, widow/widower treatment of income
- Example of a monthly contribution for cost of care
- Additional deductions from income
- Miller Trust-Income Cap States
- Income guidelines for married couples
- What is considered income?
- Documentation that will verify income
- Rental property income
- Self-employment/business income
- Veterans Benefits
- Report all Changes to income and health insurance premiums
- You must apply for all income that you are entitled to receive

Chapter 7
–Ongoing Requirements After A Case Has Been Opened

After your case has been opened and there are questions that come up that you are unclear about, it is wise to call your Medicaid representative. They are there to help you. Sometimes a phone call can clear up a lot of anxieties that you are experiencing unduly. It is best to be well informed. The Medicaid representative will give you the answers, or at least get back to you at a later date with the answer to your questions.

Changes to income and health insurance premiums

Once your Medicaid case has been opened, there are a few times during the year that you will be asked for certain information. Social Security usually gets an increase. Pensions may increase or decrease and, health insurance premiums change. You have a responsibility to report any changes in income and health insurance premiums to the agency when they occur. The Agency needs to know changes timely (usually within 10 days). Towards the end of the year letters may be sent to you requesting that you send verification of your new social security amount (to the agency) by a specified date. This is often referred to as the cost of living change or increase (also known as COLA). The reason for this is so the Medicaid representative can recalculate your monthly cost share to the nursing home. You will be sent in writing the new amount of your cost share and the nursing home will be sent a copy of the new monthly share amount as well.

Recertification/re-application/re-determination

Recertification/re-application/re-determination are all terms used by different states for periodic updates of income and resources. While doing our research on the information from state to state we determined that the time line for this process differed. Some states require Recertification every six months and some states require the process once a year. Some states allow you to send the completed Recertification to the agency via the mail, and other states require that you come in to the agency to complete the Recertification. Of course, like the application someone representing the patient may appear for the Recertification.

*   *   *

You will be required to:

- Complete the Recertification forms in ink and sign the back.
- Enclose a recent copy of the bank statement for each account (not 36 months of statements).
- Include recent cash values of life insurance for each policy.
- Verify current income and health insurance premiums.

*   *   *

Community spouses will not be required to verify their resources but will be required to verify income from all sources. Verification could be income tax returns, 1099 statements, bank letters or bank statements describing interest income. The income tax return would be a good source to verify self-employment income.

You may be notified at the case opening that you will have a certain period of time to transfer resources (such as bank accounts, ownership of life insurance policies, and deeds) to the community spouse. The Medicaid representative will more than likely follow-up to see that this has been done at Recertification.

It is a good idea to keep a copy of the completed Recertification form. It will remind you of the Recertification process. You will know what to expect when you are required to complete it again. Medicaid will compare the accounts listed on the current and previous Recertification form. They are updating account balances and looking for verification of changes.

If the nursing home patient should receive an inheritance, settlement, lump sum, or windfall, verification of the amount received should be sent to the Medicaid representative immediately. An example would be a copy of a letter, which accompanies the check, or a copy of the check. Generally, lump sum payments are considered as income in the month received and then they are counted as a resource in any subsequent month. Immediately check with your Medicaid representative for a directive on to how to proceed.

Fair hearing for ongoing cases

If the department of social services has denied your ongoing medical assistance, you have the right to request a fair hearing. Often, the telephone number and information regarding the fair hearing process is on the back of the discontinuance or denial letter sent to you. After you have requested the fair hearing you will be notified of the date, time and location of the fair hearing. Attending the fair hearing will be a fair hearing officer, a Medicaid representative and yourself (it would be a good idea to have someone help you with this). You will be given the opportunity to state your position, and the Medicaid representative will state their position. The fair hearing officer will make a determination and notify you and the agency by mail of the decision rendered. The amount of time needed to make a decision will vary.

Keep the Medicaid Representative Informed

Those of you who are representing family members, friends and loved ones in the nursing home please remember that all correspondence from the Medicaid Representative will be sent to you. If you are planning on moving, changing phone numbers, going away for the winter, etc. you must inform the Medicaid Representative. It is wise to put it in writing so that a copy can be placed in the file.

You want to move your parents

Your parent/parents are in a nursing home and are receiving Medicaid in another state, and you want to move them closer to your home. Of course, the first thing to do is make the necessary arrangements with a nursing home in your area to admit your parent/parents. They will help and guide you through the transition. Your Medicaid case would close in the former state. You would need to apply for Medicaid in the state in which you are moving your parent/parents. If you have already been through the Medicaid process, you should be familiar with the requirements. You will need to contact your local Medicaid office and speak to a Medicaid representative. You will be sent the appropriate paperwork to complete the Medicaid application process.

If you follow the path through this book we think that you will be pleasantly surprised. The application process doesn't have to be as overwhelming as you think it will be. We are sure that this book will help take the confusion out of the process and give you clear direction.

Summary

- Changes to income and health insurance premiums.
- Recertification/re-application/re-determination for on going benefits.
- Fair hearings for on-going cases.
- Keep the Medicaid Representative informed.
- You want to move your parents.

* * *

Appendix A
–Medicaid Application
Documentation Checklist

Did I remember to:

_____Complete the application in ink.

_____Answer all questions.

_____Read the back of the application form.

_____Sign and date the back of the application forms.

Did I remember to include?

_____Permanent documentation such as birth certificate, social security card, marriage certificate, death certificate, etc.

_____Copies of Medicare and health insurance cards.

_____Copy of Power of Attorney paperwork.

_____Verification of all sources of income.

_____The 36 months of bank records for all open and closed accounts.

_____The 60 months of financial records if there is a Trust

_____Copies of life insurance policies.

_____Copies of burial agreements, verification of cemetery plot.

_____Copies of deeds and current tax information for Real Estate owned.

_____Copies of titles or registrations for vehicles owned.

_____Copies of medical bills for the three months prior to going.

_____An explanation of resources.

Appendix B
–Recertification/Re-application Checklist

Before I send the recertification/re-application form back to the Medicaid Representative did I remember to:

_____Call my Medicaid Representative if I have questions about the form or the required paperwork.

_____Verify income-such as copies of my social security award letter, gross pension statement, copy of my recent bank statement showing my direct deposit for income.

_____Verify my current monthly health insurance premium amount such as a copy of my cancelled check or a copy of the bill stating the current amount.

_____Verify my current resource amount-such as a current bank statement for all open accounts.

_____Verify dividends received-copies of stubs or statements from financial institutions for stocks, insurance dividends, etc.

_____Verify income from all sources for community spouse-such as income tax statements, statements from financial institutions, etc.

_____Answer all questions on the recertification/re-application form.

_____Sign and date the back of the form.

Appendix C
–Rights and Responsibilities

YOU HAVE RIGHTS

- You have the right to apply or reapply any time you wish for any assistance programs
- You have the right to receive help completing the application form.
- You have a right to know the name of your Medicaid Representative
- You have the right to be told in writing why your application was approved or denied.
- You have a right to know in writing when any changes are made to your case.
- You have the right to be treated with courtesy, dignity, and respect.
- You have the right to have an agency conference to talk about your case.
- You have a right to request a fair hearing if you disagree with the agency's determination
- You have a right to review any information used to determine your eligibility and the amount you are required to pay.

You Have Responsibilities

- You have the responsibility to complete and sign the application form and verify all eligibility factors.
- You have the responsibility to give complete and accurate facts so eligibility can be determined correctly.
- You have the responsibility to report any changes as soon as they happen. This includes changes to income, changes to health insurance premiums, etc.
- You have the responsibility to apply for any other benefits you may be entitled to, such as pensions. You must apply for Medicare Part B, if not already receiving coverage.
- You have the responsibility to provide social security numbers for each household member.

Appendix D
–State Agencies on Aging

Alabama Commission on Aging
RSA Plaza, Suite 470
770 Washington Avenue
Montgomery, AL 36130-1851
(334) 242-5743
Fax: (334) 242 5594

Alaska Commission on Aging
Division of Senior Services
Department of Administration
Juneau, AK 99811-0209
(907) 465-3250
Fax: (907) 465-4716

Arizona Aging and Adult Administration
Department of Economic Security
1789 West Jefferson Street-#950A
Phoenix, AZ 85007
(602) 542-4446
Fax: (602) 542-6575

Arkansas Division Aging and Adult Services
Arkansas Dept of Human Services
PO Box 1437, Slot 1412
1417 Donaghey Plaza South
Little Rock, AR 72203-1437
(501) 682-2441
Fax: (501) 682-8155

California Department of Aging
1600 K Street
Sacramento, CA 95814
(916) 322-5290
Fax: (916) 324-1903

Colorado Aging and Adult Services
Department of Social Services
110-16th Street, Suite 200
Denver, CO 80202-4147
(303) 620-4147
Fax: (303) 620-4191

Connecticut Division of Elderly Services
25 Sigourney Street, 10th Floor
Hartford, CT 06106-5033
(860) 424-5277
Fax: (860) 424-4966

Delaware Division of Services for Aging and Adults with Physical Disabilities
Department of Health and Social Services
1901 North DuPont Highway
New Castle, DE 19720
(302) 577-4791
Fax: (302) 577-4793

District of Columbia Office on Aging
One Judiciary Square-9th Floor
441 Fourth Street, NW
Washington, DC 20001
(202) 724-5622
Fax: (202) 724-4979

Department of Elder Affairs
Building B-Suite 152
4040 Esplanade Way
Tallahassee, FL 32399-7000
(904) 414-2000
Fax: (904) 414-2004

Georgia Division of Aging Services
Department of Human Resources
2 Peachtree Street North E.36th Floor
Atlanta, GA 30303-3176
(404) 657-5258
Fax: (404) 657-5285

Guam Division of Senior Citizens
Department of Public Health & Social Services
PO Box 2816
Agana, Guam 96910
011-671-475-0263
Fax: 671-477-2930

Hawaii Executive Office on Aging
250 South Hotel Street, Suite 109
Honolulu, HI 96813-2831
(808) 586-0100
Fax: (808) 586-0185

Idaho Commission on Aging
PO Box 83720
Boise, ID 83720-0007
(208) 334-3833
Fax: (208) 334-3033

IL Department on Aging
421 East Capitol Avenue, Suite 100
Springfield, IL 62701-1789
(217) 785-2870
Chicago Office: (312) 814-2916
Fax: (217) 785-4477

Indiana Bureau of Aging and In-Home Services

Division of Disability, Aging and Rehabilitative Services
Family and Social Services Administration
402 West Washington Street, #W454
PO Box 7083
Indianapolis, IN 46207-7083
(317) 232-7020
Fax: (317) 232-7867

Iowa Department of Elder Affairs
Clemens Building, 3rd Floor
200 Tenth Street
Des Moines, IA 50309-3609
(515) 281-4646
Fax: (515) 281-4036

Kansas Department on Aging
New England Building
503 SOUTH Kansas Avenue.
Topeka, KS 66603-3404
785-296-4986
Fax: (785) 296-0256

Kentucky Office of Aging Services
Cabinet for Families and Children
Commonwealth of Kentucky
275 East Main Street
Frankfort, KY 40621
(502) 564-6930
Fax: (502) 564-4595

Louisiana Governor's Office of Elderly Affairs
PO Box 80374
Baton Rouge, LA 70898-0374
(504) 342-7100
Fax: (504) 342-7133

Maine Bureau of Elder and Adult Services
Department of Human Services
35 Anthony Avenue
State House-Station #11
Augusta, ME 04333
(207) 624-5335
Fax: (207) 624-5361

Maryland Department of Aging
State Office Building, Room 1007
301 West Preston Street
Baltimore, MD 21201-2374
(410) 767-1100
Fax: (410) 333-7943

Massachusetts Executive Office of Elder Affairs
One Ashburton Place, 5th Floor
Boston, MA 02108
(617) 727-7750
Fax: (617) 727-9368

Michigan Office of Services to the Aging
611 West Ottawa, North Ottawa Tower, 3rd Floor
PO Box 30676
Lansing, MI 48909
(517) 373-8230
Fax: (517) 373-4092

Minnesota Board on Aging
444 Lafayette Road
Street Paul, MN 55155-3843
(612) 297-7855
Fax: (612) 296-7855

Mississippi Division of Aging and Adult Services
750 North State Street
Jackson, MS 39202
(601) 359-4925
Fax: (601) 359-4370

Missouri Division on Aging
Department of Social Services
PO Box 1337
615 Howerton Court
Jefferson City, MO 65102-1337
(573) 751-3082
Fax: (573) 751-8687

Montana Senior and Long Term Care Division
Department of Public Health & Human Services
PO Box 4210
111 Sanders, Room 211
Helena, MT 59620
(406) 444-7788
Fax: (406) 444-7743

**Nebraska Department of Health and
Human Services Division on Aging**
PO Box 95044
1343 M Street
Lincoln, NE 68509-5044
(402) 471-2307
Fax: (402) 471-4619

Nevada Division for Aging Services
Department of Human Resources
State Mail Room Complex
3416 Goni Road, Building D
Carson City, NV 89706
Phone: (775) 687-4210
Fax: (775) 687-4264

New Hampshire Division of Elderly and Adult Services
State Office Park South
129 Pleasant Street, Brown Bldg. #1
Concord, NH 03301
(603) 271-4680
Fax: (603) 271-4643

Department of Health and Senior Services
New Jersey Division of Senior Affairs
P.O Box 807
Trenton, New Jersey 08625-0807
(609) 588-3141
(800) 792-8820
Fax: (609) 588-3601

New Mexico State Agency on Aging
La Villa Rivera Building
228 East Palace Avenue Ground Floor
Santa Fe, NM 87501
(505) 827-7640
Fax: (505) 827-7649

New York State Office for the Aging
2 Empire State Plaza
Albany, NY 12223-1251
(800) 342-9871
(518) 474-5731
Fax: (518) 474-0608

North Carolina Department of Health and Human Services Division of Aging
2101 Mail Service Center
Raleigh, NC 27699-2101
(919) 733-3983
Fax: (919) 733-0443

North Dakota Department of Human Services Aging Services Division
600 South 2nd Street, Suite 1C
Bismarck, ND 58504
(701) 328-8910
Fax: (701) 328-8989

North Mariana Islands CNMI Office on Aging
PO Box 2178
Commonwealth of the Northern Mariana Islands
Saipan, MP 96950
(670) 233-1320/1321
Fax: (670) 233-1327/0369

Ohio Department of Aging
50 West Broad Street-9th Floor
Columbus, OH 43215-5928
(614) 466-5500
Fax: (614) 466-5741

Oklahoma Aging Services Division
Department of Human Services
PO Box 25352
312 NORTH E. 28th Street
Oklahoma City, OK 73125
(405) 521-2281 or 521-2327
Fax: (405) 521-2086

OR Senior and Disabled Services Division
500 Summer Street, NORTH E., 2nd Floor
Salem, OR 97310-1015
(503) 945-5811
Fax: (503) 373-7823

Palau State Agency on Aging
Republic of Palau
Koror, PW 96940
9-10-288-011-680-488-2736
Fax: 9-10-288-680-488-1662 or 1597

Pennsylvania Department of Aging
Commonwealth of Pennsylvania
555 Walnut Street, 5th floor
Harrisburg, PA 17101-1919
(717) 783-1550
Fax: (717) 772-3382

Commonwealth of Puerto Rico
Governor's Office of Elderly Affairs
Call Box 50063
Old San Juan Station, PR 00902
(787) 721-5710, 721-4560, 721-6121
Fax: (787) 721-6510

Rhode Island Department of Elderly Affairs
160 Pine Street
Providence, RI 02903-3708
401 277-2858
Fax: (401) 277-2130

American Samoa Territorial Administration on Aging
Government of American Samoa
Pago Pago, American Samoa 96799
011-684-633-2207
Fax: 011-864-633-2533 or 633-7723

SC Office of Senior and Long Term Care Services
Department of Health and Human Services
PO Box 8206
Columbia, SC 29202-8206
(803) 898-2501
Fax: (803) 898-4515

South Dakota Office of Adult Services and Aging
Richard F. Kneip Building
700 Governors Drive
Pierre, SD 57501-2291
(605) 773-3656
Fax: (605) 773-6834

Tennessee Commission on Aging
Andrew Jackson Building. 9th floor,
500 Deaderick Street,
Nashville, Tennessee 37243-0860
(615) 741-2056
Fax: (615) 741-3309

Texas Department on Aging
4900 North Lamar, 4th Floor
Austin, TX 78751-2316
(512) 424-6840
Fax: (512) 424-6890

Utah Division of Aging & Adult Services
Box 45500
120 North 200 West
Salt Lake City, UT 84145-0500
(801) 538-3910
Fax: (801) 538-4395

Vermont Department of Aging and Disabilities
Waterbury Complex
103 South Main Street
Waterbury, VT 05671-2301
(802) 241-2400
Fax: (802) 241-2325

Virginia Department for the Aging
1600 Forest Avenue, Suite 102
Richmond, VA 23229
(804) 662-9333
Fax: (804) 662-9354

Virgin Islands Senior Citizen Affairs
Virgin Islands Department of Human Services
Knud Hansen Complex, Building A
1303 Hospital Ground
Charlotte Amalie, VI 00802
(340) 774-0930
Fax: (340) 774-3466

Washington Aging and Adult Services Administration
Department of Social & Health Services
PO Box 45050
Olympia, WA 98504-5050
(360) 493-2500
Fax: (360) 438-8633

West Virginia Bureau of Senior Services
Holly Grove-Building 10
1900 Kanawha Boulevard East
Charleston, WV 25305
(304) 558-3317
Fax: (304) 558-0004

Wisconsin Bureau of Aging and Long Term Care Resources
Department of Health and Family Services
PO Box 7851
Madison, WI 53707
(608) 266-2536
Fax: (608) 267-3203

Wyoming Office on Aging
Department of Health
117 Hathaway Building-Room 139
Cheyenne, WY 82002-0710
(307) 777-7986
Fax: (307) 777-5340

Appendix E
–Long Term Care Ombudsmen

Ombudsmen investigate and resolve complaints and insure that individuals receive fair treatment while residing in nursing homes and other long term care facilities. The address and phone number for the Long-Term Care Ombudsman program for your state is listed below.

Alabama
RSA Plaza, Suite 470
770 Washington Avenue
Montgomery, AL 36130
(334) 242-5743
Fax: (334) 242-5594

Alaska
Older Alaskans Commission
3601 C Street, Suite 260
Anchorage, AK 99503-5209
(907) 563-6393
Fax: (907) 561-3862

Arkansas
DIV. AGING & ADULT SERVICES
State Long-Term Care Ombudsman
P.O Box 1437, Slot 1412
Little Rock, AR 72201-1437
(501) 682-2441
Fax: (501) 682-8155

Arizona
State Long-Term Care Ombudsman
AGING AND ADULT ADMINISTRATION
Department of Economic Security
1789 West Jefferson-950A
Phoenix, AZ 85007
(602) 542-4446
Fax: (602) 542-6575

California
State Long-Term Care Ombudsman
Department of Aging
1600 K Street
Sacramento, CA 95814
(916) 3232-6681
Fax: (916) 323-7299

Colorado
State Long-Term Ombudsman
The Legal Center
455 Sherman Street Suite 130
Denver, CO 80203
(303) 722-0300
Fax: (303) 722-0720

Connecticut
Department on Aging
25 Sigourney Street-10th Floor
Hartford, CT 06106-5033
(860) 424-5200 ext. 5221
Fax: (860) 424-4966

Delaware
Delaware Services for Aging-Disabled
Health & Social Services
Oxford Building, Suite 200
256 Chapman Road
Newark, DE 19702
(302) 453-3820 x 46
Fax:(302) 453-3836

District of Columbia
AARP-Legal Counsel for the Elderly
601 E Street, North West 4th Floor, Bldg. A
Washington, DC 20049
(202) 434-2140

Florida
Florida State LTC Ombudsman Council
Holland Building, Rm. 270
600 South Calhoun Street
Tallahassee, FL 32301
(850) 488-6190
Fax: (850) 488-5657

Georgia
Division of Aging Services
2 Peachtree Street NW, 36th Floor
Suite 36-385
Atlanta, GA 30303-3176
(404) 657-5319
Fax: (404) 657-5285

Hawaii
Executive Office on Aging
Office of the Governor
250 South Hotel Street, Suite 107
Honolulu, HI 96813-2831
(808) 586-0100
Fax: (808) 586-0185

Idaho
Office on Aging
PO Box 83720
700 West Jefferson, Room 108
Boise, ID 83720-0007
(208) 334-3833
Fax: (208) 334-3033

Illinois
Illinois Department on Aging
421 East Capitol Avenue Suite 100
Springfield, IL 62701-1789
(217) 785-3143
Fax: (217) 524-4477

Indiana
Indiana Division of Aging & Rehabilitative Services
PO Box 7083-W454
402 West Washington Street
Indianapolis, IN 46207-7083
(317) 232-1750
Fax: (317) 232-7867

Iowa
Iowa Department of Elder Affairs
Clemens Building
200 10th Street, 3rd Floor
Des Moines, IA 50309-3609
515-281-8643
Fax: 515-281-4036

Kansas
Office of the State Long-Term Care Ombudsman
610 SW 10th Street, 2nd Floor
Topeka, KS 66612-1616
785-296-3017
Fax: 785-296-3916

Kentucky
Division of Family/Children Services
275 E Main St, 5th Fl W
Frankfort, KY 40621
502-564-6930
Fax: 502-564-4595

Louisiana
Governor's Office of Elderly Affairs
412 North 4th Street, 3rd Floor
PO Box 80374
Baton Rouge, LA 70802
(225) 342-7100
Fax: (225) 342-7144

Maine
Maine State Long Term Care Ombudsman Program
1 Weston Court
PO Box 126
Augusta, ME 04332
(207) 621-1079
Fax: (207) 621-0509

Maryland
OFFICE ON AGING
State Office Building, Room 1007
301 West Preston Street
Baltimore, MD 21201
(410) 767-1074
Fax: (410) 333-7943

Massachusetts
Executive Office of Elder Affairs
1 Ashburton Place, 5th floor
Boston, MA 02108-1518
(617) 727-7750
Fax: (617) 727-9368

Michigan
Citizens for Better Care
6105 West Street Joseph Highway, Suite 211
Lansing, MI 48917-3981
517-886-6797
Fax: 517-886-6349
In-state toll free: (800) 292-7852

Minnesota
OFFICE OF OMBUDSMAN FOR OLDER MINNESOTANS
85 East Seventh Place, Suite 280
Street Paul, MN 55155-3843
(651) 296-0382
Fax: (651) 297-5654

Mississippi
Div of Aging & Adult Services
750 North State Street
Jackson, MS 39202
(601) 359-4929
Fax: (601) 359-4970

Missouri
DIVISION ON AGING
Department of Social Services
PO Box 1337
615 Howerton Court
Jefferson City, MO 65102-1337
(573) 526-0727
Fax: (573) 751-8687

Montana
OFFICE ON AGING
Department of Health and Human Services
Senior & LTC Division
PO Box 4210
111 Sanders
Helena, MT 59604-4210
(406) 444-4077
Fax: (406) 444-7743

Nebraska
DEPARTMENT ON AGING
PO Box 95044
301 Centennial Mall-South
Lincoln, NE 68509-5044
(402) 471-2306
Fax: (402) 471-4619

Nevada
DIVISION FOR AGING SERVICES
Department of Human Resources
340 North 11th Street, Suite 203
Las Vegas, NV 89101
(702) 486-3545
Fax: (702) 486-3572

New Hampshire
Division of Elderly & Adult Services
129 Pleasant Street
Concord, NH 03301-3857
(603) 271-4375
Fax: (603) 271-4771

New Jersey
PO Box 807
Trenton, NJ 08625-0807
(609) 588-3614
Fax: (609) 588-3365

New Mexico
STATE AGENCY ON AGING
228 East Palace Avenue
Santa Fe, NM 87501
(505) 827-7640
Fax: (505) 827-7649

New York
OFFICE FOR THE AGING
2 Empire State Plaza
Agency Bldg. #2
Albany, NY 12223-0001
(518) 474-7329
Fax: (518) 474-7761

North Carolina
DIVISION OF AGING
693 Palmer Drive
Caller Box 29531
Raleigh, NC 27626-0531
(919) 733-8395
Fax: (919) 733-0443

North Dakota
AGING SERVICES DIVISION, DHHS
600 South 2nd Street, Suite 1C
Bismarck, ND 58504
(701) 328-8910
Fax: (701) 328-8989

Ohio
DEPARTMENT OF AGING
50 West Broad Street-9th Fl
Columbus, OH 43215-5928
(614) 644-7922
Fax: (614) 466-5741

Oklahoma
AGING SERVICES DIVISION, DHS
312 NORTH E. 28th Street, Suite 109
Oklahoma City, OK 73105
(405) 521-6734
Fax: (405) 521-2086

Oregon
Office of the Long Term Care Ombudsman
3855 Wolverine NE, Suite 6
Salem, OR 97310
(503) 378-6533
Fax: (503) 373-0852

Pennsylvania
DEPARTMENT OF AGING
555 Walnut Street, 5th Floor
PO Box 1089
Harrisburg, PA 17101
(717) 783-7247
Fax: (717) 783-3382

Puerto Rico
GOV'S OFFICE FOR ELDER AFFAIRS
Call Box 50063, Old San Juan Station
San Juan, Puerto Rico 00902
(787) 725-1515
Fax: (787) 721-6510

Rhode Island
ALLIANCE FOR BETTER LONG-TERM CARE
422 Post Road,
Suite 204
Warwick, RI 02888
(401) 785-3340
Fax: (401) 785-3391

South Carolina
Division on Aging
1801 Main Street
PO Box 8206
Columbia, SC 29202-8206
(803) 253-6177
Fax: (803) 253-4173

South Dakota
OFFICE OF ADULT SVCS & AGING
700 Governors Drive
Pierre, SD 57501-2291
(605) 773-3656
Fax: (605) 773-6834

Tennessee
COMMISSION ON AGING
Andrew Jackson Building, 9th Floor
500 Deaderick Street
Nashville, TN 37243-0860
(615) 741-2056
Fax: (615) 741-3309

Texas
DEPARTMENT ON AGING
4900 North Lamar Blvd., 4th Floor
PO Box 12786
Austin, TX 78751-2316
(512) 424-6840
Fax: (512) 424-6890

Utah
DIV OF AGING & ADULT SVS
Dept. Of Social Services
120 North 200 West, Room 401
Salt Lake City, Utah 84103
(801) 538-3910
Fax: (801) 538-4395

Vermont
Vermont Legal Aid, Inc.
PO Box 1367
Burlington, VT 05402
(802) 863-5620
Fax: (802) 863-7152

Virginia
Virginia Association of
Area Agencies on Aging
530 East Main Street, Suite 428
Richmond, Virginia 23219
(804) 644-2923
Fax: (804) 644-5640

Washington
South King County Multi-Services Center
1200 South 336th Street
PO Box 23699
Federal Way, WA 98093
(253) 838-6810
Fax: (253) 874-7831

West Virginia
COMMISSION ON AGING
1900 Kanawha Blvd. East
Charleston, WV 25305-0160
(304) 558-3317
Fax: (304) 558-0004

Wisconsin
BOARD ON AGING AND LONG TERM CARE
214 North Hamilton Street
Madison, WI 53703-2118
(608) 266-8945 Ext. DIR
Fax: (608) 261-6570

Wyoming
WYOMING SENIOR CITIZENS, INC.
756 Gilchrist
PO Box 94
Wheatland, WY 82201
(307) 322-5553
Fax: (307) 322-3283

Appendix F
–State Medicaid Offices

ALABAMA MEDICAID OFFICES

BIRMINGHAM

85 Bagby Drive, Room 302
Birmingham, AL 35209-3707
(205) 912-2100
County Served: Jefferson County

DECATUR

2119 Westmeade Drive SW
(PO Box 1728, ZIP 35602-1728)
Decatur, AL 35603-1050
(205) 584-4100
Counties Served: Cullman, Jackson, Madison, Marshall, Morgan

DOTHAN

2652 Fortner Street, Suite 4
Dothan, AL 36305-3203
(334) 702-3100
Counties Served: Barbpir, Coffee, Covington, Cremsjaw, Dale, Geneva, Henry, Houston, Pike

FLORENCE
214 East College Street
Florence, AL 35630-5437
Mail to: PO Box 895
Florence, AL 25631-0895
(205) 740-6100
Counties Served: Colbert, Franklin, Lauderdale, Lawrence, Limestone, Marion, Winston

GADSDEN
200-DW Meighan Blvd.
Gadsden, AL 35901-3200
Mail to: PO Box 35
Gadsden, AL 35902-0035
(205) 549-7700
Counties Served: Blount, Calhoun, Cherokee, Cleburne, DeKalb, Etowah, Saint Clair

MOBILE
4367 Downtowner Loop N Suite D
Mobile, AL 36609-5558
(334) 304-2150
Counties Served: Baldwin, Conecuh, Escambia, Mobile, Washington

MONTGOMERY
501 Dexter Avenue
Montgomery, AL 36104-3744
Mail to: PO Box 5624
Montgomery, AL 36103-5624
(334) 242-4065
Counties Served: Autauga, Bullock, Elmore, Montgomery

AUBURN-OPELIKA
1716 Catherine Court
Suite 1A
Auburn, AL 36830-9938
(334) 502-5446
Counties Served: Chambers, Clay, Coosa, Lee, Macon, Randolph, Russell, Tallapoosa, Talladega

SELMA
1120 Water Avenue
Selma, AL 36701-4619
Mail to: PO Box 2539
Selma, AL 36702-2539
(334) 418-6600
Counties Served: Bibb, Butler, Chilton, Choctaw, Clarke, Dallas, Lowndes, Marengo, Monroe, Perry, Wilcox

TUSCALOOSA
2110 McFarland Blvd. E.-Suite G
Tuscaloosa, AL 35404-5822
Mail to: PO Box 020706
Tuscaloosa, AL 35402-0706)
(205) 391-6760
Counties Served: Fayette, Greene, Hale, Lamar, Pickens, Shelby, Sumter, Tuscaloosa, Walker

ALASKA MEDICAID OFFICES

ANCHORAGE APA OFFICE
235 E. 8th Avenue, Suite 300
Anchorage, Alaska 99501
(907) 269-6000

ANCHORAGE DISTRICT OFFICE
400 Gambell Street, Suite 101
Anchorage, Alaska 99501
(907) 269-6599

BETHEL DISTRICT OFFICE
406 Ridgecrest Drive
PO Box 365
Bethel, Alaska 99559-0365
(907) 543-2686 or (800) 478-2686

COASTAL FIELD OFFICE
3601 C Street, Suite 410
PO Box 240249
Anchorage, Alaska 99524-0249
(907) 269-8950 or (800) 478-4372

EAGLE RIVER JOB CENTER
11723 Old Glenn Highway, #B-4
Eagle River, Alaska 99577-7595
(907) 694-7006

FAIRBANKS DISTRICT OFFICE
675 7th Street, Station G
Fairbanks, Alaska 99701
(907) 451-2850 or (800) 478-2850

HOMER DISTRICT OFFICE
601 East Pioneer Avenue, Suite 122
Homer, Alaska 99603
(907) 235-6132

JUNEAU DISTRICT OFFICE
10002 Glacier Highway, Suite 201
Juneau, Alaska 99801
(907) 465-3551 or (800) 478-3551

KENAI PENINSULA JOB CENTER
11312 Kenai Spur Highway, #2
Kenai, Alaska 99611
(907) 283-2900 or (800) 478-9032

KETCHIKAN DISTRICT OFFICE
2030 Sea Level Drive, Suite 301
Ketchikan, Alaska 99901-1955
(907) 225-2135 or (800) 478-2135

KODIAK DISTRICT OFFICE
307 Center Street
Kodiak, Alaska 99615
(907) 486-3783 or (888) 480-3783

KOTZEBUE DISTRICT OFFICE
PO Box 1210
Kotzebue, Alaska 99752
(907) 442-3451

MAT-SU DISTRICT OFFICE
855 W Commercial Drive
Wasilla, Alaska 99654
(907) 376-3903 or (800) 478-7778

MULDOON ONE STOP
1251 Muldoon Road, Suite 111B
Anchorage, Alaska 99504
(907) 269-0000

NOME DISTRICT OFFICE
PO Box 2110
Nome, Alaska 99762
(907) 443-2237 or (800) 478-2236

SEAPA/SPECIALIZED MEDICAID
10002 Glacier Highway, Suite 105
Juneau, Alaska 99801
(907)465-3537 or (800) 478-3537

SITKA DISTRICT OFFICE
201 Katlian Street, #107
Sitka, Alaska 99835
(907) 747-8234 or (800) 478-8234

AMERICAN SAMOA
Department of Health
American Samoa Government
Pago Pago, AS 96799
(684) 633-5237
Fax: 011 (684) 633-4240

ARIZONA LONG TERM CARE OFFICES

CASA GRANDE
500 North Florence Street
Casa Grande, AZ 85222
(520) 421-1500
Fax: (520) 836-6828

CENTRAL OFFICE
801 East Jefferson Street
Phoenix, AZ 85034
(602) 417-4000
Fax: (602) 256-9305
MAIL DROP-2300-Program Support
MAIL DROP-2600-Field Operations l

CHINLE
PO Box 1942
Chinle, AZ 86503
(520) 674-5439
Toll Free: 1-888-800-3804
Fax: (520) 674-5494

COTTONWOOD
One North Main Street
Cottonwood, AZ 86326
(520) 634-8101
Fax: (520) 634-8007

FLAGSTAFF
3480 East Route 66
Flagstaff, AZ 86004
(520) 527-4104
Toll Free: (800) 342-0567
Fax: (520) 527-1686

GLENDALE
2830 West Glendale Avenue
Suite 19, Suite 34 & Suite 8
Phoenix, AZ 85051
(602) 417-6000
Fax: (602) 864-0854 (Financial)
Fax: (602) 995-0635 (Medical)

GLOBE/MIAMI
Cobre Valle Plaza
2250 Highway 60
Suite H
Miami, AZ 85539-9700
(520) 425-3165
Fax: (520) 425-7316

KIDSCARE
920 East Madison
Suite E.
Mail Drop 500
Phoenix, AZ 85034
(602) 417-6800
(602) 417-5437
Toll Free: 1-877-764-5437
Fax: (602) 417-6850
Fax: (602) 417-6851

KINGMAN
519 East Beale Street
Suite 150
Kingman, AZ 86401
(520) 753-2828
Fax: (520) 753-6995

LAKE HAVASU CITY
285 South Lake Havasu Avenue.
Lake Havasu City, AZ 86403
(520) 453-5100
Fax: (520) 453-6057

MESA
460 North Mesa Drive
Suite 101
Mesa, AZ 85201
(602) 417-6400
Fax: (480) 644-0878

PHOENIX
4440 North 36th Street
Phoenix, AZ 85018
(602)-417-6200
Fax: (602) 957-4068 (Financial)
Fax: (602) 224-0479 (Medical)

PHOENIX SOUTH (TANNER BUILDING)
700 East Jefferson Street
Mail Drop 600
Phoenix, AZ 85034
(602) 417-6600
Fax: (602) 417-6650 (Financial)
Fax: (602) 417-6660 (Medical)

PRESCOTT
1570 Willow Creek Road
Prescott, AZ 86301
(520) 778-3968
Toll Free: (800) 824-2656
Fax: (520) 778-1232 (Financial)

SHOW LOW
580 East Old Linden Road
Suite 3
Show Low, AZ 85901
(520) 537-1515
Toll Free: 1-877-537-1515
Fax: (520) 537-1822

SIERRA VISTA
484 East Wilcox Drive
Sierra Vista, AZ 85635
(520) 459-7050
Fax: (520) 459-0702

SSI-MAO (TANNER BUILDING)
700 E. Jefferson Street
Phoenix, AZ 85034
(602) 417-6672
Toll Free: (800) 528-0142
Fax: (602) 417-6995

TUCSON-FINANCIAL
Magdalena Building
110 South Church Avenue
Suite 2070
Tucson, AZ 85701
(520) 205-8600
Toll Free: (800) 824-2656
Fax: (520) 205-8709
PO Box 3049
Tucson, AZ 85702

TUCSON-MEDICAL
Tuluca Building
110 South Church Avenue
Suite 3250
Tucson, AZ 85701
(520) 205-8600
Toll Free: (800) 824-2656
Toll Free: (800) 423-9132 (Director's Office)
Fax: (520) 205-8708 (Medical)
Fax: (520) 205-8706 (Director's Office)
PO Box 3049
Tucson, AZ 85702

YUMA
3850 West 16th Street
Suite B
Yuma, AZ 85364
(520) 782-0776
Fax: (520) 782-2894

ARKANSAS DEPARTMENT OF HUMAN SERVICES
COUNTY OFFICES

ARKANSAS
100 Court Square
Dewitt, AR 72042
(870) 946-4519

ARKANSAS
PO Box 270
203 South Leslie
Stuttgart, AR 72160
(870) 673-3597

ASHLEY
PO Box 190
201 West Lincoln
Hamburg, AR 31646
(870) 853-9816

BAXTER
PO Box 408
204 Bucher Drive
Mountain Home, AR 72654
(870) 425-6011

BENTON
1206 Southeast J Street
Bentonville, AR 72712
(501) 273-9011

BOONE
PO Box 1096
2126 Capps Road
Harrison, AR 72601
(870) 741-6107

BRADLEY
PO Box 509
902 Halligan
Warren, AR 71671
(870) 226-5878

CALHOUN
PO Box 1068
136 Archer
Hampton, AR 71744
(870) 798-4201

CARROLL
PO Box 425
304 Hailey Road
Berryville, AR 72616
(870) 423-3351

CHICOT
PO Box 71
1736 Highway 65 & 82 South
Lake Village, AR 71653
(870) 265-3821

CLARK
PO Box 968
602 South 10th Street
Arkadelphia, AR 71923
(870) 246-9886

CLAY
PO Box 366
187 North, 2nd Street
Piggott, AR 72454
(870) 598-2282

CLAY
1007 Ada Street
Corning, AR 72422
(870) 857-6544

CLEBURNE
PO Box 1140
1521 West Main
Heber Springs, AR 72543
(501) 362-3298

CLEVELAND
PO Box 465
501 Main Street
Pison, AR 7166S5
(870) 325-6218

COLUMBIA
PO Box 1109
601 East University
Magnolia, AR 71754
(870) 234-4190

CONWAY
PO Box 228
#2 Bruce Street
Morrilton, AR 72110
(501) 354-2418

CRAIGHEAD
2920 McClellan Drive
Jonesboro, AR 72401
(870) 972-1732

CRAWFORD
704 Cloverleaf Circle
Van Buren, AR 72956
(501) 474-7595

CRITTENDEN
250 Shoppingway
Memphis, AR 72301
(870) 732-5170

CROSS
PO Box 572
803 East Highway 64
Wynne, AR 72396
(870) 238-8553

DALLAS
1202 West 3rd Street
Fordyce, AR 71742
(870) 352-5115

DESHA
Box 111
200 North Main Street
McGehee, AR 71654
(870) 222-4144

DREW
PO Box 449
210 South Main
Monticello, AR 71657
(870) 367-683S

FAULKNER
PO Box 310
1000 E, Slebenmorgan Rd
Conway, AR 72033
(501) 730-9900

FRANKLIN
800 West Commercial
Ozark, AR 72949
(501) 667-2379

FULTON
PO Box 650
201 Byron Road
Salem, AR 72576
(870) 895-3309

GARLAND
115 Market Street
Hot Springs, AR 71901
(510) 321-2583

GRANT
PO Box 158
16 Opportunity Drive
Sheridan, AR 72150
(870) 942-5151

GREENE
PO Box 839
809 Goldsmith Road
Paragould, AR 72451
(870) 236-8723

HEMPSTEAD
116 North Laurel
Hope, AR 71801
(870) 777-8656

HOT SPRING
PO Box 813
2505 Pine Bluff Street
Malvern, AR 72104
(501) 332-2718

HOWARD
PO Box 1740
North Main
Nashville, AR 71852
(870) 845-4334

INDEPENDENCE
1750 Myers Street
Batesville, AR 72501-7393
(870) 698-1876

INDEPENDENCE
PO Box 2517
Highway 25 North
Batesville, AR 72501-7393
(870) 793-6876

IZARD
PO Box 65
620 East Main Street
Melbourne, AR 72556
(870) 368-4318

JACKSON
PO Box 658
3rd & Hazel Street
Newport, AR 72112
(870) 523-9820

JEFFERSON
PO Box 5670
1222 West 6th
Pine Bluff, AR 71601
(870) 534-4200

JOHNSON
PO Box 1636
900 South Rogers Avenue
Clarksville, AR 72830
(501) 754-2355

LAFAYETTE
PO Box 970
Highway 29 North
Lewisville, AR 71845
(870) 921-4283

LAWRENCE
PO Box 69
North West 4th Street
Walnut Ridge, AR 72476
(870) 886-2408

LEE
PO Box 309
772 West Chestnut Street
Marianna, AR 72360
(870) 295-2597

LINCOLN
101 West Wiley Street
Star City, AR 71667
(870) 628-4105

LITTLE RIVER
90 Waddell Street
Ashdown, AR 71822
(870) 898-5155

LOGAN
17 West McKeen Street
Paris, AR 72855-3228
(501) 963-2783

LOGAN
390 East 2nd Street
Booneville, AR 72927-3703
(501) 675-3091

LONOKE
PO Box 260
100 Park Street
Lonoke, AR 72086
(501) 676-5643

MADISON
P0 Box 128
1013 North College Avenue
Huntsville, AR 72740
(501) 738-2161

MARION
PO Box 447
36 Main Street
Yellville, AR 72687
(870) 449-4058

MILLER
4323 Jefferson Street
Texarkana, AR 71854
(870) 773-0563

MISSISSIPPI
218 North First Street
Blytheville, AR 72315-2802
(870) 763-7093

MISSISSIPPI
437 South Country Club Road
Osceola, AR 72370-4207
(870) 563-5234

MONROE
PO Box 354
Highway 302 North
Clarendon, AR 72029-2791
(870) 747-3329

MONROE
3011/2 North New Orleans
Brinkley, AR 72021-2813
(870) 734-1445

MONTGOMERY
PO Box 445
205 Highway 27 South
Mount Ida, AR 71957-0445
(870) 867-3184

NEVADA
PO Box 292
West 1st Street
Prescott, AR 71857-0292
(870) 887-6626

NEWTON
PO Box 452
Co-Op Building
Jasper, AR 72641-0452
(870) 446-2237

OUACHITA
PO Box 718
222 Van Buren Street North West
Camclen, AR 71711-3931
(870) 836-8166

PERRY
403 Houston Avenue
Perryville, AR 72126-9539
(501) 889-5105

PHILLIPS
PO Box 277
104 D'Anna Place
Helena, AR 72342-0439
(870) 338-8391

PIKE
PO Box 200
East 13th Street
Murfreesboro, AR 71958-0200
(870) 285-3111

POINSETT
PO Box 526
510-A South Illinois Street
Harrisburg, AR 72432-0526
(870) 578-5491

POLK
606 Pine Street
Mena, AR 71953-0807
(501) 393-3100

POPE
701 North Denver
Russellville, AR 72801-3403
(501) 968-5596

PRAIRIE
PO Box 356
4 Market Street
DeValls Bluff, AR 72041-0356
(870) 998-2581

PULASKI SOUTH
PO Box 2620
1105 Martin Luther King Junior Drive
Little Rock, AR 72203-2620
(501) 682-9231

PULASKI NORTH
PD Box 5791
1900 East Washington Avenue
North Little Rock, AR 72119-5791
(501) 682-0100

PULASKI SOUTH WEST
PO Box 8916
6801 Baseline Road
Little Rock, AR 72219-8916
(501) 371-1100

PULASKI EAST
1424 East Second Street
Little Rock, AR 72201
(501) 371-1300

PULASKI JACKSONVILLE
PO Box 626
2636 West Main Street
Jacksonville, AR 72078
(501) 371-1200

RANDOLPH
1408 Pace Road
Pocahontas, AR 72455-4307
(870) 992-4475

SALINE
PO Box 608
1603 Edison Avenue
Benton, AR 72018-0608
(501) 315-1600

SCOTT
PO Box 840
South Highway 71B
Waldron, AR 72958-0840
(501) 637-4141

SEARCY
PO Box 279
350 School Street
Marshall, AR 72650-0279
(870) 448-3153

SEBASTIAN
616 Garrison Avenue
Fort Smith, AR 72901-2598
(501) 782-4555

SEVIER
108 Town North
West Collin Raye Drive
Professional Building A
DeQueen, AR 71832-2007
(870) 642-2623

SHARP
PO Box 159
Highway 167 North
Ash Flat, AR 72513-0159
(870) 994-7358

SAINT FRANCIS
PO Box 899
1200 East Broadway
Forrest City, AR 72336
(870) 633-1242

STONE
HC 71, Box 180
Mountain View, AR 72560-9638
(870) 269-4321

UNION
123 West 18th Street
El Dorado, AR 71730-7098
(870) 862-6631

VAN BUREN
Route 6, Box 260-1
Clinton, AR 72031-0126
(501) 745-4192

WASHINGTON
4044 Frontage Road
Fayetteville, AR 72703-2084
(501) 521-1270

WASHINGTON
4171 North Crossover Road
Fayetteville, AR 72703
(501) 442-4029

WHITE
608 Rodgers Drive
Searcy, AR 72143-4199
(501) 268-8696

WOODRUFF
PO Box 493
1200 Highway 33 North
Augusta, AR 72006-0493
(870) 347-2537

YELL
PO Box 277
818 M Street, Highway 10 East
Danville, AR 72833-0277
(501) 495-2723

CALIFORNIA COUNTY DEPARTMENTS OF SOCIAL SERVICES

ALAMEDA
401 Broadway, Rm. 500
Oakland, CA 94607
510-268-2100
case inquiries: (510) 268-2002
Fax: (510) 268-7366

ALPINE
75 Diamond Valley Rd
Markleeville, CA 96120
(530) 694-2235
Fax: (530) 694-2252

AMADOR
108 Court St
Jackson, CA 95642-2379
(209) 223-6550
Fax: (209) 267-1504

BUTTE
42 County Center Drive
Oroville, CA 95965
(530) 538-7572
Fax: (530) 534-5745

CALAVENUERAS
Government Center
891 Mountain Ranch Road
San Andreas, CA 95249
(209) 754-6452
Fax: (209) 754-6724

COLUSA
251 East Webster Street
Colusa, CA 95932
(530) 458-0250
Fax: (530) 458-0492

CONTRA COSTA
40 Douglas Drive
Martinez, CA 94553
(925) 313-1500
Fax: (925) 313-1575

DEL NORTE
880 North Crest Street
Crescent City, CA 95531
(707) 464-3191

EL DORADO
3057 Briw Road
Placerville, CA 95667
(530) 642-7300
Fax: (530) 626-9060

FRESNO
4455 East Kings Canyon Road
Fresno, CA 93750-0001
(559) 453-6407
Fax: (559) 453-3782

GLENN
420 East Laurel
Willows, CA 95988
(530) 934-6514
Fax: (530) 934-6521

HUMBOLDT
929 Koster Street
Eureka, CA 95501
(707) 445-6103
case inquiries: (707) 445-6106
Fax: (707) 441-5600

IMPERIAL
2995 South Fourth Street, Suite 105
El Centro, CA 92243
(760) 337-6880
Fax: (760) 337-5716

INYO
155 East Market Street
Independence, CA 93526
Mail to: Drawer A
Independence, CA 93526
(760) 878-0247
Fax: (760) 878-0266

KERN
100 East California Avenue
Bakersfield, CA 93302
(661) 631-6000
Fax: (661) 631-6631

KINGS
1200 South Drive
Hanford, CA 93230
(559) 582-3241 ext 2202
Fax: (559) 584-2749

LAKE
15975 Anderson Ranch Parkway
Lower Lake, CA 95457
(707) 995-4200
Fax: (707) 995-4294

LASSEN
720 Richmond Road
Susanville, CA 96130
(530) 251-8152
Fax: (530) 251-8370

LOS ANGELES
Department of Children and Family Services
425 Shatto Place
Los Angeles, CA 96130
(213) 351-5602
Fax: (213) 252-8437

MADERA
629 East Yosemite Avenue
Madera, CA 93638
(559) 675-7841
Fax: (559) 675-7603

MARIN
20 North San Pedro Road, Suite 2028
San Rafael, CA 94903
(415) 499-6924
Fax: (415) 499-3791

MARIPOSA
5186 Highway 49 North
Mariposa, CA 95338
(209) 966-3609
Fax: (209) 966-5943

MENDOCINO
747 South State Street
Ukiah, CA 95482
(707) 463-7700
Fax: (707) 463-7804

MERCED
2115 West Wardrobe Avenue
Merced, CA 95341
(209) 385-3000
Fax: (209) 383-6925

MODOC
120 North Main Street
Alturas, CA 96101
(530) 233-6501
Fax: (530) 233-2136

MONO
PO Box 576
Bridgeport, CA 93517
(760) 932-7291
Fax: (760) 932-5287

MONTEREY
1000 South Main Street, Suite 208
Salinas, CA 93901
(831) 755-4400
Fax: (831) 755-8477

NAPA
2261 Elm Street
Napa, CA 94559-3721
(707) 253-4279
Fax: (707) 253-6172

NEVADA
950 Maidu Avenue
Nevada City, CA 95959
(530) 265-1340
Fax: (530) 265-7062

ORANGE
888 North Main Street
Santa Ana, CA 92701
(714) 541-7700
Fax: (714) 541-7811

PLACER
11519 B Avenue
Auburn, CA 95603
(530) 889-7610
Case inquiries (530) 889-7613
Fax: (530) 889-7128

PLUMAS
270 County Hospital Road
Quincy, CA 95971
(530) 283-6350
Fax: (530) 283-6368

RIVERSIDE
4060 County Circle Drive
Riverside, CA 92503
(909) 358-3000
Case inquiries (909) 358-3300
Fax: (909) 358-3036

SACRAMENTO
3701 Branch Center Road, Room 213
Sacramento, CA 95827-3822
(916) 875-6091
Fax: (916) 875-5553

SAN BENITO
1111 San Felipe Road, Suite 206
Hollister, CA 95023
(408) 637-5336
Fax: (408) 637-9754

SAN BERNARDINO
385 North Arrowhead Avenue, 5th Floor
San Bernardino, CA 92415-5128
(909) 387-5040
Fax: (909) 387-3081

SAN DIEGO
1700 Pacific Highway, Room 207
San Diego, CA 92101
(619) 515-6555
Fax: (619) 515-6556

SAN FRANCISCO
PO Box 7988
San Francisco, CA 94120
(415) 557-6541
Fax: (415) 431-9270

SAN JOAQUIN
102 South San Joaquin Street
Stockton, CA 95201-3006
(209) 468-1000
Fax: (209) 468-1985

SAN LUIS OBISPO
3433 South Higuera Street
San Luis Obispo, CA 93403-8119
(805) 781-1600
Fax: (805) 781-1846

SAN MATEO
400 Harbor Boulevard
Belmont, CA 94002
(650) 595-7500
Fax: (650) 595-7516

SANTA BARBARA
234 Camino Del Remedio
Santa Barbara, CA 93110
(805) 681-4400
Fax: (805) 681-4403

SANTA CLARA
1725 Technology Drive
San Jose, CA 95110-1360
(408) 441-5100
Fax: (408) 436-1337

SANTA CRUZ
1000 Emeline Street
Santa Cruz, CA 95060
(831) 454-4045
Case inquiries (831) 454-4150
Fax: (831) 454-4642

SHASTA
375 Lake Boulevard
Redding, CA 96049-6005
(530) 225-5777
Case inquiries (530) 225-5613
Fax: (530) 225-5361

SIERRA
PO Box 1019
Loyalton, CA 96118
(530) 993-6720
Fax: (530) 993-6741

SISKIYOU
311 Fourth Street, Room 4
Yreka, CA 96097
(530) 841-2700
Fax: (530) 841-2791

SOLANO
PO Box 4090
Mail Stop 3-200
Fairfield, CA 94533-0677
(707) 553-5311
Fax: (707) 421-6618

SONOMA
2550 Paulin Drive
Santa Rose, CA 95402-1539
(707) 527-2715
Case inquiries (707) 527-2663
Fax: (707) 565-5890

STANISLAUS
251 East Hackett Road
Modesto, CA 95353-0042
(209) 558-2500
Fax: (209) 558-2558

SUTTER
PO Box 1535
Yuba City, CA 95992
(530) 822-7230
Fax: (530) 822-7255

TEHAMA
22840 Antelope Boulevard
Red Bluff, CA 96080
(530) 527-1911
Fax: (530) 527-5410

TRINITY
1 Industrial Park Way
Weaverville, CA 96093-1470
(530) 623-1265
Fax: (530) 623-1250

TULARE
5957 South Mooney Boulevard
Visalia, CA 93277
(559) 737-4682
Fax: (559) 737-4692

TUOLUMNE
20075 Cedar Road North
Sonora, CA 95370
(209) 533-5711
Fax: (209) 533-5714

VENTURA
505 Poli Street
Ventura, CA 93001
(805) 652-7602
Fax: (805) 652-7571

YOLO
120 West Main Street
Woodland, CA 95695
(530) 661-2750
Fax: (530) 661-2728

YUBA
6000 Lindhurst Avenue, Suite 504
Marysville, CA 95901
(530) 749-6311
Fax: (530) 749-6281

COLORADO DEPARTMENTS OF SOCIAL SERVICES COUNTY OFFICES

ADAMS
7190 Colorado Blvd
Commerce City, CO 80022
(303) 287-8831
(303) 227-2106

ALAMOSA
610 State Street (physical)
Alamosa, CO 81101
Mail to: PO Box 1310
Alamosa, CO 81101
(719) 589-2581
Fax: (719) 589-9794

ARAPAHOE
1690 West Littleton Blvd
Littleton, CO 80120-2069
(303) 795-4850
Fax: (303) 795-4861

ARCHULETA
449 San Juan
Pagosa Springs, CO 81147
PO Box 240
Pagosa Springs, CO 81147
(970) 264-2182
Fax: (970) 264-2186

BACA
772 Colorado Street
Springfield, CO 81073
(719) 523-4131
Fax: (719) 523-4820

BENT
215 2nd Street
Las Animas, CO 81054
PO Box 326
(719) 456-2620
Fax: (719) 456-2945

BOULDER
3400 Broadway
Boulder, CO 80304
(303) 441-1000
Fax: (303) 441-1289

CHAFFEE
Mail to: PO Box 1007
Salida, CO 81201
641 West 3rd Street
Salida, CO 81201
(719) 539-6627
Fax: (719) 539-6430

CHEYENNE
PO Box 146
Cheyenne Wells, CO 80810
51 South 1st
Cheyenne Wells, CO 80810
(719) 767-5629
Fax: (719) 767-5101

CLEAR
Courthouse
Georgetown, CO 80444
Mail to: PO Box 2000
Georgetown, CO 80444
(303) 569-3251, x371
Fax: (303) 679-2443

CONEJOS
Courthouse
Conejos, CO 81129
Mail to: PO Box 68
Conejos, CO 81129
(719) 376-5455
Fax: (719) 376-2389

COSTILLA
123 Gasper Street
San Luis, CO 81152
Mail to: PO Box 249
San Luis, CO 81152
(719) 672-4131
Fax: (719) 672-4141

CROWLEY
601 Main
Ordway, CO 81063
Mail to: PO Box 186
Ordway, CO 81063
(719) 267-3546
Fax: (719) 267-4072

CUSTER
205 South 6th Street
Westcliffe, CO 81252
Mail to: PO Box 929
Westcliffe, CO 81252
(719) 783-2371
Fax: (719) 783-2885

DELTA
Courthouse Annex, 560 Dodge
Delta, CO 81416
(970) 874-2030
Fax: (970) 874-2068

DENVER
1200 Federal Blvd.
Denver, CO 80204-3221
(720) 944-3666
Fax: (720) 944-3096

DOLORES
420 North Main, Courthouse
Dove Creek, CO 81324
Mail to: PO Box 485
Dove Creek, CO 81324
(970) 677-2250
Fax: (970) 677-2815

DOUGLAS
101 Third Street
Castle Rock, CO 80104
(303) 688-4825
Fax: (303) 688-0292

EAGLE
500 Broadway Street
Eagle, CO 81631
Mail to: PO Box 660
Eagle, CO 81631
(970) 328-8840
Fax: (970) 328-6227

ELBERT
Mail to: PO Box 6
Simla, CO 80835
325 Pueblo Avenue
Simla, CO 80835
(719) 541-2369
Fax: (719) 541-9505

EL PASO
105 North Spruce
Colorado Springs, CO 80905
PO Box 2692
Colorado Springs, CO 80901
(719) 444-5532
Fax: (719) 444-5598

FREMONT
172 Justice Center Road
Canon City, CO 81212
(719) 275-2318
Fax: (719) 275-5206

GARFIELD
2014 Blake Avenue
Glenwood Springs, CO 81602
PO Box 580
Glenwood Springs, CO 81602-0580
(970) 945-9191
Fax: (970) 928-0465

GILPIN
2960 Dory Hill Road, Suite 100
Black Hawk, CO 80403-8780
(303) 582-5444
Fax: (303) 582-5798

GRAND
620 Hemlock
Hot Sulphur Springs, CO 80451
Mail to: PO Box 204
Hot Sulphur Springs, CO 80451
(970) 725-3331
Fax: (970) 725-3696

GUNNISON
225 North Pine Street, Suite A
Gunnison, CO 81230
(970) 641-3244
Fax: (970) 641-3738

HINSDALE
225 North Pine Street, Suite A
Gunnison, CO 81230
(970) 641-3244
Fax: (970) 641-3738

HUERFANO
121 West 6th Street
Walsenburg, CO 81089
(719) 738-2810
Fax: (719) 738-2549

JACKSON
Mail to: PO Box 204
Hot Sulpher Springs, CO 80451
(970) 723-4750
Fax: (970) 723-4706

JEFFERSON
900 Jefferson County Parkway
Golden, CO 80401-6010
(303) 277-1388
Fax: (303) 271-4444

KIOWA
Courthouse
1305 Goff Street
Eads, CO 81036
PO Box 187
Eads, CO 81036
(719) 438-5541
Fax: (719) 438-5370

KIT CARSON
252 South 14th Street
Burlington, CO 80807
(719) 346-8732
Fax: (719) 346-8066

LAKE
112 West 5th Street
Leadville, CO 80461
Mail to: PO Box 884
Leadville, CO 80461
(719) 486-2088
Fax: (719) 486-4164

LA PLATA
1060 East Second Avenue
Durango, CO 81301
(970) 382-6150
Fax: (970) 274-2208

LARIMER
1501 Blue Spruce Drive
Fort Collins, CO 80524-2000
(970) 498-6300
Fax: (970) 498-7987

LAS ANIMAS
204 South Chestnut Street
Trinidad, CO 81082
(719) 846-2276
Fax: (719) 846-4269

LINCOLN
Courthouse
103 3rd Avenue
Hugo, CO 80821
PO Box 37
Hugo, CO 80821
(719) 743-2404
Fax: (719) 743-2879

LOGAN
508 South 10th Avenue, Suite 2
Sterling, CO 80751
Mail to: PO Box 1746
Sterling, CO 80751
(970) 522-2194
Fax: (970) 521-0853

MESA
2952 North Avenue
Grand Junction, CO 81502
PO Box 20000-5035
Grand Junction, CO 81502
(970) 241-8480
Fax: (970) 248-2702

MINERAL
1015 6th Street
Del Norte, CO 81132
Mail to: PO Box B
Del Norte, CO 81132
(719) 657-3381
Fax: (719) 657-4013

MOFFAT
595 Breeze Street
Craig, CO 81625
(970) 824-8282
Fax: (970) 824-9552

MONTEZUMA
109 West Main, Room 203
Cortez, CO 81321
(970) 565-3769
Fax: (970) 565-8526

MONTROSE
107 South Cascade
Montrose, CO 81402
Mail to: PO Box 216
Montrose, CO 81402
(970) 249-3401
Fax: (970) 249-3402

MORGAN
231 Ensign Street, Admin Bldg.
Fort Morgan, CO 80701
PO Box 220
Fort Morgan, CO 80701
(970) 542-3530
Fax: (970) 542-3544

OTERO
Courthouse, 3rd & Colorado
La Junta, CO 81050
PO Box 494
La Junta, CO 81050
(719) 383-3100
Fax: (719) 383-3150

OURAY
541 4th Street
Ouray, CO 81427
Mail to: PO Box M
Ouray, CO 81427
(970) 325-4437
Fax: (970) 325-4438

PARK
288 Main Street
Bailey, CO 80421
Mail to: PO Box 1193
Bailey, CO 80421
(719) 838-0082
Fax: (719) 836-7286

PHILLIPS
246 South Interocean
Holyoke, CO 80734
(970) 854-2280
Fax: (970) 854-3637

PITKIN
0405 Castle Creek Road, #8
Aspen, CO 81611
(970) 920-5350
Fax: (970) 920-5360

PROWERS
1001 South Main
Lamar, CO 81052
PO Box 1157
Lamar, CO 81052
(719) 336-7486
Fax: (719) 336-7198

PUEBLO
212 West 12th Street
Pueblo, CO 81003
(719) 583-6160
Fax: (719) 583-6377

RIO BLANCO
555 Main Street, Room 102
Meeker, CO 81641
Mail to: PO Box 688
Meeker, CO 81641
(970) 878-5011
Fax: (970) 878-5796

RIO GRANDE
1015 6th Street
Del Norte, CO 81132
Mail to: PO Box B
Del Norte, CO 81132
(719) 657-3381
Fax: (719) 657-4013

ROUTT
136 6th Street
Steamboat Springs, CO 80477
Mail to: PO Box 772790
Steamboat Springs, CO 80477
(970) 879-1540
Fax: (970) 870-5260

SAGUACHE
605 Christy Avenue
Saguache, CO 81149
Mail to: PO Box 215
Saguache, CO 81149
(719) 655-2537
Fax: (719) 655-0206

SAN JUAN
1557 Greene Street
Silverton, CO 81433
(970) 387-5631

SAN MIGUEL
333 West Colorado Avenue
Telluride, CO 81435
Mail to: PO Box 96
Telluride, CO 81435
(970) 728-4411
Fax: (970) 728-4412

SEDGWICK
106 West 1st
Julesburg, CO 80737
Mail to: PO Box 27
Julesburg, CO 80737
(970) 474-3397
Fax: (970) 474-9881

SUMMIT
37 County Road 1005
Frisco, CO 80443
Mail to: PO Box 869
Frisco, CO 80443
(970) 668-4100
Fax: (970) 668-4115

TELLER
740 Highway 24
Woodland Park, CO 80866-9033
Mail to: PO Box 9033
Woodland Park, CO 80866-9033
(719) 687-6268
Fax: (719) 687-0429

WASHINGTON
875 East 1st Street
Akron, CO 80720
(970) 345-2238
Fax: (970) 345-2237
(888) 844-2238

WELD
315 North 11th Avenue
Greeley, CO 80631
PO Box A
Greeley, CO 80631
(970) 352-1551
Fax: (970) 353-5215

YUMA
340 South Birch Street
Wray, CO 80758-1814
(970) 332-4877
Fax: (970) 332-4978

CONNECTICUT DEPARTMENT OF SOCIAL SERVICES

CENTRAL OFFICE:
Connecticut Department of Social Services
25 Sigourney Street
Hartford, CT 06106
Information and Referral: (800) 842-1508
Toll free TDD/TTY line: (800) 842-4524

NORTH CENTRAL REGION:

Hartford
3580 Main Street
Hartford, CT 06120-1187
(860) 723-1111
Towns Served: Bloomfield, East Granby, Granby, Hartford, Newington, Rocky Hill, Suffield, West Hartford, Wethersfield, Windsor, Windsor Locks

Bristol
45 North Main Street
Bristol, CT 06010-8111
(860) 314-6558
Towns Served: Avon, Bristol, Burlington, Canton, Farmington, Plymouth, Simsbury, Southington

New Britain
270 Lafayette Street
New Britain, CT 06053-4174
(860) 612-3457
Towns Served: Berlin, New Britain, Plainville

Manchester
699 East Middle Turnpike
Manchester, CT 06040-3744
(860) 647-5901 or
(860) 647-5905
Towns Served: Andover, Bolton, East Hartford, East Windsor, Ellington, Enfield, Glastonbury, Hebron, Manchester, Marlborough, Somers, South Windsor, Stafford, Tolland, Vernon

SOUTH CENTRAL REGION:

New Haven
194 Bassett Street
(203) 974-8245
Towns Served: Ansonia, Bethany, Branford, Derby, East Haven, Hamden, Milford, New Haven, North Branford, North Haven, Orange, Seymour, Shelton, West Haven, Woodbridge

Meriden
55 West Main Street
Meriden, CT 06450-4117
(203) 630-6060
Towns Served: Meriden, Wallingford

Middletown
117 Main Street Extension
Middletown, CT 06457-3843
(860) 704-3111
Towns Served: Chester, Clinton, Cromwell, Deep River, Durham, East Haddam, East Hampton, Essex, Guilford, Haddam, Killingworth, Lyme, Madison, Middlefield, Middletown, Old Lyme, Old Saybrook, Portland, Westbrook

EASTERN REGION:

Norwich
279 Main Street
Norwich, CT 06360-5876
(860) 823-5050
Towns Served: Bozrah, Brooklyn, Canterbury, Colchester, Eastford, East Lyme, Franklin, Griswold, Groton, Killingly, Lebanon, Ledyard, Lisbon, Montville, New London, North Stonington, Norwich,

Plainfield, Pomfret, Preston, Putnam, Salem, Sprague, Sterling, Stonington, Thompson, Voluntown, Waterford, Woodstock

Windham/Willimantic
670-676 Main Street
Willimantic, CT 06226-2702
(860) 465-3547
Towns Served: Ashford, Chaplin, Columbia, Coventry, Hampton, Mansfield, Scotland, Union, Willington, Windham, Willimantic

SOUTH WEST REGION:

Bridgeport
925 Housatonic Avenue
Bridgeport, CT 06606-5700
(203) 551-3000
Towns Served: Bridgeport, Easton, Fairfield, Monroe, Stratford, Trumbull

Norwalk
7 Concord Street
South Norwalk, CT 06854-3705
(203) 855-2774
Towns Served: New Canaan, Norwalk, Weston, Westport, Wilton

Stamford
1642 Bedford Street
Stamford, CT 06905-4731
(203) 251-9311
Towns Served: Darien, Greenwich, Stamford

NORTH WEST REGION:

Waterbury
249 Thomaston Avenue
Waterbury, CT 06702-1397
(203) 597-4001
Towns Served: Beacon Falls, Cheshire, Middlebury, Naugatuck, Oxford, Prospect, Southbury, Waterbury, Watertown, Wolcott

Danbury
405 Main Street
Danbury, CT 06810-4783
(203) 207-8980
Towns Served: Bethel, Bridgewater, Brookfield, Danbury, New Fairfield, New Milford, Newtown, Redding, Ridgefield, Sherman

Torrington
62 Commercial Boulevard, Suite 1
Torrington, CT 06790-9983
(860) 496-6960
Towns Served: Barkhamsted, Bethlehem, Canaan, Colebrook, Cornwall, Goshen, Hartland, Harwinton, Kent, Litchfield, Morris, New Hartford, Norfolk, North Canaan, Roxbury, Salisbury, Sharon, Thomaston, Torrington, Warren, Washington, Winchester, Woodbury

DELAWARE HEALTH AND SOCIAL SERVICES

NEW CASTLE COUNTY:

Appoquinimink State Service Center
120 Silver Lake Road,
Middletown, DE 19709
(302) 378-5770

Belvedere State Service Center
310 Kiamensi Road
Wilmington, DE 19804
(302) 995-8545

Claymont State Service Center
3301 Green Street
Claymont, DE 19703
(302) 798-2870

Delaware State Service Center
500 Rogers Road
New Castle, DE 19720
(302) 577-2970

Floyd I. Hudson State Service Center
501 Ogletown Road
Newark, DE 19711
(302) 368-6700

North East State Service Center
1624 Jessup Street
Wilmington, DE 19802
(302) 577-3150

Winder Laird Porter State Service Center
509 West 8th Street
Wilmington, DE 19801
(302) 577-3400

KENT COUNTY:

James W. Williams State Service Center
805 River Road
Dover, DE 19901
(302) 739-5301

Milford State Service Center Campus:

Milford State Service Center
11-13 Church Avenue
Milford, DE 19963
(302) 422-1300

Milford Annex
13 South Front Street
Milford, DE 19963
(302) 422-1560

Milford Draper Building
10-12 North Church Street
Milford, DE 19963
(302) 422-1400

Milford Walnut Street Building
18 North East Walnut Street
Milford, DE 19963
(302) 422-1386

SUSSEX COUNTY:

Bridgeville State Service Center
Cannon Street
Bridgeville, DE 19933
(302) 337-8261

Edward West Pyle State Service Center
Omar-Roxana Road
Frankford, DE 19945
(302) 732-9501

Laurel State Service Center
Mechanics Street
Laurel, DE 19956
(302) 856-5223

Georgetown State Service Center
546 South Bedford Street
Georgetown, DE 19947
(302) 856-5574

Anna C. Shipley State Service Center
350 Virginia Avenue.
Seaford, DE 19973
(302) 628-2000

DISTRICT OF COLUMBIA

Neighborhood Services Centers:

HEADQUARTERS
645 H. Street, North East
(202) 698-4357, (202) 724-5506

ANACOSTIA CENTER
2100 MLK, Jr. Avenue, South East
(202) 645-4597, (202) 645-4520, (202) 645-4614

CAPITOL EAST CENTER
1325 Independence Avenue, South East
(202) 698-3748

CAPITOL VIEW CENTER
5929 East Capitol Street, South East
(202) 645-4518

CONGRESS HEIGHTS CENTER
4001 South Capitol Street, South East
(202) 645-4525
60 Florida Avenue, North East
(202) 576-6000

NORTH WEST, KENNEDY STREET CENTER
508 Kennedy Street,
(202) 576-7268

NORTH EAST SERVICE CENTER
3917 Minnesota Avenue, North East
(202) 724-4080

FLORIDA MEDICAID OFFICES

AREA 1:
6425 Pensacola Blvd, Bldg. 2-1
Pensacola, Florida 32305-1701
(805) 494-5840/SunCom 690-5840
Fax: (850) 494-5843/SunCom 690-5843

AREA 2:
Area 2a
651 West 14th Street, #K
Panama City, Florida 32401
(850) 872-7690
Fax: (850) 747-5456
Counties Served: Holmes, Jackson, Washington, Bay, Guld, and Franklin
Area 2b
2639 North Monroe Street, Suite 104-B
Tallahassee, Florida 32303-4094
(850) 921-8474
Fax: (850) 921-0394
Counties Served: Calhoun, Gadsden, Liberty, Leon, Wakulla, Jefferson, Madison, and Taylor

AREA 3:
Area 3a
1130 North East 16th Avenue
Gainesville, Florida 32601-4557
(352) 955-5192
Fax: (352) 955-7164
Counties Served: Hamilton, Suwannee, Columbia, Lafayette, Gilchrist, Dixie, Levy, Alachua, Union, Bradford, and Putnam
Area 3b **
2441 West Silver Spring Blvd
Ocala, Florida 34475
(352) 732-1349
Fax: (352) 732-3076
Counties Served: Marion, Citrus, Sumter, Hernando, and Lake

AREA 4:

Area 4a

Duval Regional Service Center

921 North Davis Street

Building A, Suite 160

Jacksonville, Florida 32209-6806

(904) 353-2100 / SunCom 826-2100

Counties Served: Nassau, Baker, Duval, Clay, and Street Johns

Area 4b

210 South Beach Street

Daytona Beach, Florida 32114-4404

(904) 238-4803

Counties Served: Flagler and Volusia

AREA 5:

11351 Ulmerton Road, Suite 100

Largo, Florida 33778-1630

(813) 588-6857 / SunCom 558-6857

Fax: (813) 588-4078 / SunCom 558-4078

AREA 6:

6800 North Dale Mabry Highway, Suite 220

Tampa, Florida 33614

(813) 871-7600 / SunCom 512-8290

Fax: (813) 871-8313/ SunCom 512-8313

AREA 7:
Area 7a
400 West Robinson Street, Suite 309 South Tower
Orlando, Florida 32801
(407) 245-0855
Counties Served: Orange, Seminole, and Osceola
Area 7b
3880 South Washington Avenue
Titusville, Florida 32780
(407) 383-2713
Counties Served: Brevard

AREA 8:
Regional Services Center
2295 Victoria Avenue, Room 309
Ft. Myers, Florida 33901
(941) 338-2370 / SunCom 748-2370
Fax: (941) 338-2642 / SunCom 748-2642
(800) 226-6735 in-state only

AREA 9:
1720 E. Tiffany Drive, Suite 201-B
West Palm Beach, Florida 33407
(561) 881-5080 / SunCom 264-5086
Fax: (561) 881-5085 / SunCom 264-5085

AREA 10:
1400 West Commercial Blvd., Suite 110
Ft. Lauderdale, FL 33309
(954) 202-3200 / SunCom 423-3200
Fax: (954) 202-3220 / SunCom 423-3220

AREA 11:
8355 North West 53rd Street
Koger Center
2nd Floor Manchester Bldg
Miami, Florida 33166
(305) 499-2100 / SunCom 429-2100
Fax: (305) 499-2022 / SunCom 429-2022

GEORGIA COUNTY OFFICES

APPLING
1204 West Parker Street
Baxley, GA 31513-0622
912-366-1010
ATKINSON
204 East Legion Avenue
PO Box 278
Pearson, GA 31642-0278
(912) 422-3242

BACON
417 South Dixon Street
PO Box 447
Alma, GA 31510-0447
(912) 632-8375

BAKER
PO 540
101 Sunset Boulevard
Newton, GA 31770-0540
(912) 734-5247

BALDWIN
154 Roberson Mill Road
PO Box 430
Milledgeville, GA 31061-0430
(912) 445-4135

BANKS
423 Evans Street
PO Box 159
Homer, GA 30547-0159
(706) 677-2272

BARROW
16 Lee Street
PO Box 546
Winder, GA 30680-0546
(770) 868-4222

BARTOW
47 Brooks Drive
PO Box 818
Cartersville, GA 30120-0818
(770) 387-3710

BEN HILL
124 South Grant Street
Fitzgerald, GA 31750-2901
(912) 426-5300

BERRIEN
301 South Jefferson Street
PO Box 5008
Nashville, GA 31639-5008
(912) 686-5568

BIBB
456 Oglethorpe Street
Macon, GA 31201-3278
(912) 751-6051

BLECKLEY
401 Peacock Street
PO Box 499
Cochran, GA 31014-0499
(912) 934-3172

BRANTLEY
104 Allen Street
PO Box 308
Nahunta, GA 31553-0308
(912) 462-6171

BROOKS
201 South Barnes Street
Quitman, GA 31643
(912) 263-7567

BRYAN
51 North Courthouse Street
PO Box 398
Pembroke, GA 31321-0398
(912) 653-2805

BULLOCH
41 Pulaski Highway
PO Box 1103
Statesboro, GA 30458-8635
(912) 871-1333

BURKE
729 West 6th Street
PO Box 390
Waynesboro, GA 30830-0390
(706) 554-7751

BUTTS
178 Kennedy Drive
Jackson, GA 30233-1187
(770) 504-2200

CALHOUN
345 Main Street
PO Box 9
Morgan, GA 31766-0009
(912) 849-2625

CAMDEN
1300 Charles Gilman Avenue
PO Box 68
Kingsland, GA 31548-0068
(912) 729-4583

CANDLER
750 South Leroy Street
PO Box 46
Metter, GA 30439-0046
(912) 685-2163

CARROLL
165 Independence Drive
Carrollton, GA 30116-9000
(770) 830-2050

CATOOSA
7195 Nashville Street
PO Box 58
Ringgold, GA 30736-0058
(706) 935-2368

CHARLTON
401 West Oak Street
PO Box 395
Folkston, GA 31537-0395
(912) 496-2527

CHATHAM
2 East Henry Street
PO Box 2566
Savannah, GA 31401-6761
(912) 651-2211

CHATTAHOOCHEE
70 McNaughton Street
PO Box 70
Cusseta, GA 31805-0070
(706) 989-3681

CHATTOOGA
302 South Commerce Street
PO Box 250
Summerville, GA 30747-0250
(706) 857-0817

CHEROKEE
105 Lamar Haley Parkway
PO Box 826
Canton, GA 30114-0826
(770) 720-3610

CLARKE
284 North Avenue
PO Box 1887
Athens, GA 30601-2280
(706) 227-7000

CLAY
202 Wilson Street
PO Box 189
Fort Gaines, GA 31751-0189
(912) 768-2511

CLAYTON
877 Battlecreek Road
Jonesboro, GA 30236-1919
(770) 473-2300

CLINCH
101 East Shirley Road
PO Box 396
Homerville, GA 31634-0396
(912) 487-5263

COBB
325 Fairground Street, SE
Marietta, GA 30060-2355
(770) 528-5000

COFFEE
1300 West Baker Highway
PO Box 1119
Douglas, GA 31533-4926
(912) 389-4286

COLQUITT
1033 Ist Street, SE
PO Box 3008
Moultrie, GA 31778-5603
(912) 890-7900

COLUMBIA
6358 Columbia Road
PO Box 340
Appling, GA 30802-0340
(706) 541-1640

COOK
1010 South Hutchinson Avenue
PO Box 634
Adel, GA 31620-0634
(912) 896-3672

COWKTA
533 Highway 29 North
Newnan, GA 30263-4735
(770) 254-7234

CRAWFORD
586 North Dugger Avenue
PO Box 97
Roberta, GA 31078-0097
(912) 836-3565

CRISP
107 West 23rd Avenue
PO Box 459
Cordele, GA 31015-3812
(912) 276-2349

DADE
50 North Bond Street
PO Box 159
Trenton, GA 30752-0159
(706) 657-7511

DAWSON
424 Highway 53
PO Box 867
Dawsonville, GA 30534-0867
(706) 265-6598

DECATUR
505 Amelia Avenue
PO Box 1077
Bainbridge, GA 31718-1077
(912) 248-2420

DEKALB
178 Sams Street
Decatur, GA 30030-4134
(404) 370-5251

DODGE
112 Plaza Lane
PO Box 4219
Eastman, GA 31023-4219
(912) 374-6760

DOOLY
205 West Union Street
PO Box 385
Vienna, GA 31092-0385
(912) 268-4111

DOUGHERTY
217 West Oglethorpe Boulevard
PO Box 3249
Albany, GA 31706-3249
(912) 430-4118

DOUGLAS
6218 Hospital Way
PO Box 1135
Douglasville, GA 30134-1944
(770) 489-3000

EARLY
626 Columbia Road
PO Box 747
Blakely, GA 31723-0747
(912) 723-4331

ECHOLS
106 Church of God Street
Statenville, GA 31648-9711
(912) 559-5751

EFFINGHAM
204 Franklin Street
PO Box 345
Springfield, GA 31329-0345
(912) 754-6471

ELBERT
121 Carey Street
PO Box 1010
Elberton, GA 30635-1010
(706) 213-2001

EMANUEL
143 North Anderson Drive
PO Box 808
Swainsboro, GA 30401-0808
(912) 289-2400

EVANS
Courthouse Annex
PO Box 578
Claxton, GA 30417-0578
(912) 739-1222

FANNIN
990 East Main Street, Suite 10
Blue Ridge, GA 30513-4534
(706) 632-2296

FAYETTE
905 Highway 85 South
PO Box 128
Fayetteville, GA 30214-0128
(770) 460-2555

FLOYD
436 Broad Street
PO Box 193
Rome, GA 30161-3054
(706) 296-6500

FORSYTH
426 Canton Road
PO Box 21
Cumming, GA 30040-2002
(770) 781-6700

FRANKLIN
1133 Hull Street
PO Box 279
Carnesville, GA 30521-0279
(706) 384-4521

FULTON
230 Peachtree Street, NW, Suite 400
Atlanta, GA 30303-1511
(404) 657-5219

GILMER
200 Kiker Street
Ellijay, GA 30540-1328
(706) 635-2361

GLASCOCK
674 West Main Street
PO Box 225
Gibson, GA 30810-0225
(706) 598-2955

GLYNN
4420 Altama Avenue, Suite 9
PO Box 400
Brunswick, GA 31520-3001
(912) 262-3200

GORDON
639 Oothcalooga Street
PO Box 217
Calhoun, GA 30701-2392
(706) 624-1200

GRADY
250 2nd Avenue, SE
PO Box 269
Cairo, GA 31728-0269
(912) 377-3154

GREENE
1951 South Main Street
PO Box 460
Greensboro, GA 30642-0460
(706) 453-2365

GWINNETT
530 North Dale Road
Lawrenceville, GA 30045-4537
(770) 995-2100

HABERSHAM
1045 Hollywood Highway
PO Box 160
Clarkesville, GA 30523-0003
(706) 754-2148

HALL
970 McEver Road
Gainesville, GA 30504-3938
(770) 453-2365

HANCOCK
Augusta Highway
PO Box 70
Sparta, GA 31087-0070
(706) 444-1203

HARALSON
21 Magnolia Street
PO Box 324
Buchannan, GA 30113-0324
(770) 646-3885

HARRIS
134 North College Street
PO Box 285
Hamilton, GA 31811-0285
(706) 628-4226

HART
469 East Howell Street
PO Box 518
Hartwell, GA 30643-0518
(706) 376-5157

HEARD
7686 US Highway 27
PO Box 385
Franklin, GA 30217-0385
(706) 675-3361

HENRY
125 Henry Parkway
McDonough, GA 30253-6636
(770) 954-2014

HOUSTON
92 Cohen Walker Drive
Warner Robins, GA 31088-2729
(912) 988-7600

IRWIN
108 North Irwin Avenue
Ocilla, GA 31774-1507
(912) 468-7406

JACKSON
456 Athens Street
PO Box 526
Jefferson, GA 30549-0526
(706) 367-3000

JASPER
144 North Warren Street
Monticello, GA 31064-1154
(706) 468-6461

JEFF DAVIS
206 East Sycamore Street
PO Box 706
Hazlehurst, GA 31539-0706
(912) 375-3942

JEFFERSON
2459 U.S Highway 1, North
PO Box 570
Louisville, GA 30434-0570
(912) 625-7259

JENKINS
500 Gray Street Extension
PO Box 808
Millen, GA 30442-0808
(912) 982-1944

JOHNSON
729 West Court Street
PO Box 500
Wrightsville, GA 31096-0500
(912) 864-4210

JONES
Highway 18, South
PO Box 192
Gray, GA 31032-0192
(912) 986-3126

LAMAR
122 Westgate Plaza
PO Box 970
Barnesville, GA 30204-0970
(770) 358-5170

LANIER
313 Roquemore Circle
Lakeland, GA 31635-1500
(912) 482-3686

LAURENS
904 Claxton Dairy Road
PO Box 68
Dublin, GA 31021-5479
(912) 275-6533

LEE
121 Fourth Street
PO Box 145
Leesburg, GA 31763-0145
912-759-3000

LIBERTY
508 North Main Street
Hinesville, GA 31313-2512
912-370-2555

LINCOLN
171 North Peachtree Street
PO Box 220
Lincohnon, GA 30817-0220
706-359-3135

LONG
Academy Street
PO Box 369
Ludowici, GA 31316-0369
912-545-2177

LOWNDES
206 South Patterson Street
Valdosta, GA 31601-5621
912-333-7054

LUMPKIN
175 Tipton Drive
Dahlonega, GA 30533-1604
706-864-1980

MACON
403 South Sumter Road
PO Box 457
Oglethorpe, GA 31068-0457
912-472-3700

MADISON
Courthouse Square, Highway 29
PO Box 176
Danielsville, GA 30633-0176
706-795-2128

MARION
Baker Street & 5th Avenue
PO Box 473
Buena Vista, GA 31803-0473
912-649-2311

MCDUFFIE
307 Greenway Street
PO Box 507
Thomson, GA 30824-0507
706-595-2946

MCINTOSH
1221 North Way
PO Box 1139
Darien, GA 31305-1139
912-437-4193

MERIWETHER
49 Gay Connector
Greenville, GA 30222-3339
706-672-4244

MILLER
69 Thompson Town Road
Colquitt, GA 31737-5204
912-758-3387

MITCHELL
90 West Oakland Avenue
PO Box 348
Camilla, GA 31730-0348
912-522-3500

MONROE
107 Martin Luther King Jr. Drive
PO Box 734
Forsyth, GA 31029-0734
912-993-3030

MONTGOMERY
130 East Spring Street
PO Box 217
Mt. Vernon, GA 30445-0217
912-583-1271

MORGAN
2005 South Main Street, Suite 100
PO Box 89
Madison, GA 30650-0089
706-343-5800

MURRAY
830 G. 1. Maddox Parkway
PO Box 1014
Chatsworth, GA 30705-1014
706-695-7315

MUSCOGEE
2100 Comer Avenue
PO Box 2627
Columbus, GA 31902-2627
706-649-7311

NEWTON
2165 Williams Street, NE
Covington, GA 30014-2447
770-784-2490

OCONEE
48 Greensboro Highway
PO Box 105
Watkinsville, GA 30677-0105
706-769-5206

OGLETHORPE
231 Union Point Street
PO Box 160
Lexington, GA 30648-1060
706-743—8152

PAULDING
145 Academy Drive
PO Box 168
Dallas, GA 30132-0168
770-443-7810

PEACH
700 Spruce Street, Wing E
PO Box 976
Fort Valley, GA 31030-0976
912-825-6428

PICKENS
255 Chambers Street
Jasper, GA 30143-1219
706-692-4701

PIERCE
621 Hendry Street
Blackshear, GA 31516-0620
912-449-6624

PIKE
606 Highway 19 South
PO Box 387
Zebulon, GA 30295-0387
770-567-8424

POLK
100 County Loop Road
PO Box 147
Cedartown, GA 30125-0147
706-749-2232

PULASKI
107 North Dooley Street
PO Box 567
Hawkinsville, GA 31036-0567
912-783-6191

PUTNAM
675 Godfrey Road
PO Box 3670
Eatonton, GA 31024-3670
706-485-4921

QUITMAN
Main Street
PO Box 68
Georgetown, GA 31754-0068
912-334-2427

RABUN
Hiawassee Street
PO Box 787
Clayton, GA 30525-0787
706-782-4283

RANDOLPH
311 North Webster Street
Cuthbert, GA 31740-1269
912-732-3742

RICHMOND
520 Fenwick Street
PO Box 2277
Augusta, GA 30903-2277
706-721-2536

ROCKDALE
975 Taylor Street, SW
Conyers, GA 30012-5357
770-388-5025

SCHLEY
103 West Oglethorpe Street
PO Box 367
Ellaville, GA 31806-0367
912-937-2591

SCREVEN
110 Singleton Avenue
PO Box 513
Sylvania, GA 30467-0513
912-564-2041

SEMINOLE
108 West 4th Street
Donalsonville, GA 31745-1514
912-524-2365

SPALDING
411 East Solomon Street
Griffin, GA 30223-3317
770-228-1386

STEPHENS
1000 East Tugalo Street
Toccoa, GA 30577-1941
706-282-4505

STEWART
Highway 27, Broad Street
PO Box 308
Lutupkin, GA 318IS-0308
912-838-4335

SUMTER
1542 East Forsyth Street
PO Box 1669
Americus, GA 31709-1669
912-931-2462

TALBOT
Jordan City Road
PO Box 96
Talbotton, GA 31827-0096
706-665-8S24

TALIAFERRO
107 Commerce Street
PO Box 3840
Crawfordville, GA 30631-0040
706-456-2339

TATTNALL
117 North Main Street
PO Box 518
Reidsville, GA 30453-0518
912-557-7721

TAYLOR
Highway 137, West
PO Box 366
Butler, GA 31006-0366
912-862-5221

TELFAIR
310 East Brewton Street
PO Box 456
McRae, GA 31055-0456
912-868-3030

TERRELL
642 Randolph Street, SE
PO Box 30
Dawson, GA 31742-0030
912-995-4005

THOMAS
438 Smith Avenue
PO Box 2740
Thomasville, GA 31799-2740
912-225-4005

TIFF
1212 Chestnut Avenue
PO Box 7550
Tifton, GA 31793-7550
912-386-3388

TOOMBS
162 Oxley Drive
PO Box 191
Lyons, GA 30436-0191
912-526-8117

TOWNS
456 North Main Street,
The Mail: PO Box 156
Hiawassee, GA 30546-0156
706-896-3524

TREUTLEN
108 Martin Luther King Jr., Drive
PO Box 625
Soperton, GA 30457-0625
912-529-3757

TROUP
504 East Depot Street
LaGrange, GA 30241-4631
706-845-4200

TURNER
336 North Street
PO Box 804
Ashburn, GA 31714-0804
912-567-4353

TWIGGS
719-A Highway 80 East
PO Box 530
Jeffersonville, GA 31044-0530
912-945-3258

UNION
301 School Circle
PO Box 220
Blairsville, GA 30514-0220
706-745-2931
Fax: (706) 745-3560

UPSON
711 North Bethel Street
Thomaston, GA 30286-3103
706-646-6043

WALKER
10056 North Highway 27
PO Box 689
Rock Spring, GA 30739-0689
706-375-0726

WALTON
I 110 East Spring Street
PO Box 927
Monroe, GA 30655-0927
770-207-4000

WARE
1200 Plant Avenue
PO Box 2048
Waycross, GA 31502-2048
912-285-6040

WARREN
224 North Legion Drive
PO Box 166
Warrenton, GA 30828-0166
706-465-3326

WASHINGTON
1124 South Harris Street
PO Box 108
Sandersville, GA 31082-0108
912-552-6021

WAYNE
1220 South 1st Street
Jesup, GA 31545-5157
912-427-5866

WEBSTER
Highway 4
PO Box 9
Preston, GA 31824-0009
912-828-6265

WHEELER
Third Avenue
PO Box 221
Alamo, GA 30411-0221
912-568-7127

WHITE
1241 Helen Highway, Suite 200
Cleveland, GA 30528-6938
706-865-3128

WHITFIELD
1142 Chattanooga Road
PO Box 1203
Dalton, GA 30722-1203
706-272-2331

WILCOX
304 Second Avenue
PO Box 246
Rochelle, GA 31079-0246
912-365-2242

WILKES
48 Lexington Avenue
PO Box 126
Washington, GA 30673-0126
706-678-2814

WILKINSON
I I I West Main Street
PO Box 526
Irwinton, GA 31042-0526
912-946-2224

WORTH
503 North Henderson Street
PO Box 527
Sylvester, GA 31791-0527
912-777-2000

GUAM

GUAM DEPARTMENT OF PUBLIC HEALTH AND SOCIAL SERVICES

Government of Guam
PO Box 2816
Agana, GU 96932
123 Chalan Kareta, Route 10
Mangilao, GU 96923
(671) 735-7399
Fax: (671) 734-5910
Per correspondence from Governor Carl T. C. Gutierrez, nursing home services are not a covered benefit under the Guam Medicaid State Plan.

Hawaii
Department of Human Services
Med-Quest Division Eligibility Offices

OAHU
Island of Oahu
PO Box 339
Honolulu, HI 96809
Long Term Care Eligibility   808-587-3521
Nursing Home Without Walls   808-832-0212

Kapolei Unit
601 Kamokila Boulevard, Rm. 415
Honolulu, HI 96707
Long Term Care Eligibility 808-692-7364

HAWAII

East Section
88 Kanoelehua Avenue, Rm. 107
Hilo, HI 96720
Long Term Care Eligibility   808-933-0339
Nursing Home Without Walls   808-933-8820

West Section
Frame 10 Building
75-5586 Ololi Road, Suite 3004
Kailua-Kona, HI 96740
Long Term Care Eligibility   808-329-3454
Nursing Home Without Walls   808-329-6855

KAUAI
4473 Pahee Street, Suite A
Lihue, HI 96766
Long Term Care Eligibility 808-241-3575
Nursing Home Without Walls   808-241-3343

MAUI
2145 Wells Street, Suite 103
Wailuku, HI 96793
Long Term Care Eligibility   808-243-5780
Nursing Home Without Walls   808-243-5125

MOLOKAI
65 Makaena Street, Rm. 110
Kaunakakai, HI 96748
Long Term Care Eligibility   808-553-3295

LANAI
Long Term Care Eligibility   808-565-7271
See Maui Office

IDAHO REGIONAL MEDICAID SERVICE CENTERS
(Including Personal Care Services)

REGION 1 COEUR D'ALENE
1250 Ironwood Drive
Suite 304
Coeur d'Alene, ID 83814
(208) 769-1567
Counties: Benewah, Bonner, Boundary, Kootenai, Shoshone

REGION 2 LEWISTON
1118 "F" Street
Lewiston, ID 83501-0182
(208) 799-4430
Counties: Clearwater, Idaho, Latah, Lewis, Nez Perce

REGION 3 CALDWELL
3402 Franklin Road
Caldwell, ID 83605-6932
(208) 454-0421
Counties: Adams, Canyon, Gem, Owyhee, Payette, Washington

REGION 4 BOISE
1720 Westgate Drive, Suite A
Boise, ID 83704
(208) 334-0940
Counties: Ada, Boise, Elmore, Valley

REGION 5 TWIN FALLS
601 Pole Line Road
Suite 3
Twin Falls, ID 83301
(208) 736-3024
Counties: Blaine, Camas, Cassia, Gooding, Jerome, Lincoln, Minidoka, Twin Falls

REGIONAL 6 POCATELLO
1070 Hiline Road
PO Box 4166
Pocatello, ID 83205-4166
(208) 235-2960

REGION 7 IDAHO FALLS
150 Shoup Avenue, Suite 19
Idaho Falls, ID 83402
(208) 528-5750
Counties: Bonneville, Clark, Custer, Fremont, Jefferson, Lemhi, Madison, Teton

ILLINOIS
LOCAL OFFICE DIRECTORY
Downstate Offices:

ADAMS (Region IV)
300 Main Street, 2nd Floor
PO Box 451
Quincy, IL 62306-0451
(217) 223-0550

ALEXANDER (Region V)
1401 Washington Avenue
Cairo, IL 62914
(618) 734-0762
(618) 734-0763
(618) 734-0764

BOND (Region V)
100 North Locust Street
Greenville, IL 62246-1535
(618) 664-0668

BOONE (Region 11)
2090 Pearl Street
Belvidere, IL 61008-0800
(815) 544-3484

BROWN (Region IV)
206 South West Cross Street
Mt. Sterling, IL 62353
(217) 773-3307, (217) 773-3308

BUREAU (Region 111)
225 Backbone Road East #2
Princeton, IL 61356-9543
(815) 875-1134, (815) 872-4331

CALHOUN (Region IV)
807 West Main Street
PO Box 220
Hardin, IL 62047-0220
(618) 576-2258

CARROLL (Region 11)
820 South Mill Road
PO Box 153
Mt. Carroll, IL 61053-0153
(815) 244-3301, (815) 244-1155

CASS (Region IV)
300 East Second Street
Beardstown, IL 62618-1225
(217) 323-4185, (217)323-4212

CHAMPAIGN (Region 111)
801 North Walnut Street
PO Box 1787
Champaign, IL 61824-1787
(217) 278-5605

CHRISTIAN (Region IV)
1100 North Cheney
PO Box 468
Taylorville, IL 62568-0468
(217) 287-7334

CLARK (Region IV)
315 South 14th Street
Marshall, IL 62441-1743
(217) 826-2541, (217) 826-5141

CLAY (Region V)
(618)-665-3391
Highway 45 & Chestnut Street
PO Drawer C
Louisville, IL 62858-0903
(618) 665-3391, (618) 665-3392

CLINTON (Region V)
1130 12th Street
Carlyle, IL 62231-1252
(618) 594-2407

COLES (Region IV)
119 West State Street
Charleston, IL 61920-1399
(217) 345-2188

CRAWFORD (Region V)
1110 North Allen Street
PO Box 656
Robinson, IL 62454-0656
(618) 544-3151

CUMBERLAND (Region IV)
200 South Indiana
PO Box 188
Toledo, IL 62468-0188
(217) 849-3541

DEKALB (Region 11)
2245 Gateway Drive
Sycamore, IL 60178-3164
(815) 756-4805

DEWITT (Region IV)
1275 Route 54 East
PO Box 438
Clinton, IL 61727-0438
(217) 935-2166

DOUGLAS (Region IV)
207 East Ficklin
PO Box 470
Tuscola, IL 61953-0470
(217) 253-3347

DUPAGE (Region 11)
146 West Roosevelt Road
Villa Oaks Office Concourse-Suite 2
Villa Park, IL 60181-3575
(630) 530-1120

EDGAR (Region IV)
206 East Court Street
Paris, IL 61944-2295
(217) 465-6491

EDWARDS (Region V)
332 Industrial Drive
PO Box 150
Albion, IL 62806-1329
(618) 445-2121

EFFINGHAM (Region IV)
925 East Fayette Avenue
PO Box 726
Effingham, IL 152401-0726
(217) 342-4160

FAYETTE (Region V)
228 West Johnson Street
Vandalia, IL 62471-2898
(618) 283-2607

FORD (Region 111)
500 West Ottawa Road
PO Box 254
Paxton, IL 60957-0254
(217) 379-2141

FRANKLIN (Region V)
1602 North Main Street
Benton, IL 62812-1900
(618) 439-4351, (618) 439-4352, (618) 439-4353, (618) 439-4354

FULTON (Region 111)
1329 North Main Street
PO Box 312
Lewistown, IL 61542-0312
(309) 547-3755

GALLATIN (Region V)
9525 Gold Hill Road
PO Box 280
Shawneetown, IL 62984-0280
(618) 269-3128, (618) 269-3129

GREENE (Region IV)
145 Walnut Street
PO Box 286
Carrollton, IL 62016-0286
(217) 942-6907, (217) 942-6908

GRUNDY (Region 11)
1715 Division Street, Suite 105
Morris, IL 60450-3100
(815) 942-3024

HAMILTON (Region V)
Route 14 East
PO Box 146
McLeansboro, IL 62859-0146
(618) 643-2313

HANCOCK (Region IV)
620 Wabash Street
Carthage, IL 62321-1444
(217) 357-3116

HARDIN (Region V)
108 North Main
PO Box 307
Elizabethtown, IL 62931-0307
(618) 287-2521, (618) 287-3491

HENDERSON (Region III)
Highway 164 East
Oquawka, IL 61469
(309) 867-3071

HENRY (Region 111)
125 West South Street, Suite 14
Kewanee, IL 61443-3741
(309) 852-5627, (309) 852-5628

IROQUOIS (Region 111)
1790 East Walnut
PO Box 341
Watseka, IL 60970-0341
(815) 432-5256, (815) 432-5257

JACKSON (Region V)
342 North Street
Murphysboro, IL 62966-2295
(618) 687-1705

JASPER (Region V)
910 South Van Buren Street
Newton, IL 62448-1727
(618) 783-2311

JEFFERSON (Region V)
414 East Main Street
PO Box 1607
Mt. Vernon, IL 62864-1607
(618) 242-1040

JERSEY (Region IV)
110 North Jefferson Street
Jerseyville, IL 62052-1726
(618) 498-2105

JO DAVIESS (Region 11)
708 South West Street
PO Box 237
Galena, IL 61036-0237
(815) 777-0718

JOHNSON (Region V)
803 Vine Street
PO Box 186
Vienna, IL 62995-0186
(618) 658-4261, (618) 658-9401, (618) 658-8182

KANE/AURORA (Region 11)
361 Old Indian Trail
Aurora, IL 60506-2430
(630) 844-7400

KANE/ELGIN (Region 11)
600 South State Street
Elgin, IL 60123-7610
(847) 931-2700

KANKAKEE (Region 11)
285 North Schuyler Avenue
PO Box 1786
Kankakee, IL 60901-1786
(815) 939-4544

KENDALL (Region 11)
1304 Game Farm Road
Yorkville, IL 60560-1497
(630) 553-7743

KNOX (Region 111)
1580 East Knox Street
Galesburg, IL 61401-5396
(309) 342-8144, (309) 342-8145, (309) 342-8146

LAKE (Region 11)
3235 West Belvidere Road
Park City, IL 60085-6017
(847) 336-5212

LASALLE (Region 111)
700 Centennial Drive
Ottawa, IL 61350-1073
(815) 443-2392

LAWRENCE (Region V)
RR 1, Box 418
Lawrenceville, IL 62439-9784
(618) 943-2334

LEE (Region 11)
201 Lincoln Statue Drive
PO Box 568
Dixon, IL 61021-0568
(815) 288-4125

LIVINGSTON (Region 111)
905 Custer Avenue
PO Box 707
Pontiac, IL 61764-0707
(815) 842-1151

LOGAN (Region IV)
1550 4th Street
PO Box 310
Lincoln, IL 62656-0310
(217) 735-2306, (217) 735-2307, (217) 735-2308

MACON (Region IV)
707 East Wood Street
PO Box 3130
Decatur, IL 62524-3130
(217) 362-6500

MACOUPIN (Region IV)
85 Carlinville Plaza
PO Box 380
Carlinville, IL 62626-0380
(217) 854-3145

MADISON/GRANITE CITY (Region V)
16 Nameoki Village Shopping Center
Granite City, IL 62040-3798
(618) 877-9200

MADISON/EAST ALTON (Region V)
608 West Saint Louis Avenue
PO Box 270
East Alton, IL 62024-0270
(618) 258-1660

MARION (Region V)
100 East McCord Street
PO Box 746
Centralia, IL 62801-0746
(618) 532-1966, 532-1967, 532-1968

MARSHALL (Region 111)
511 School Street
Henry, IL 61537-1236
(309) 364-2376

MASON (Region 111)
323 West Main Street
Havana, IL 62644-1194
(309) 543-3329

MASSAC (Region V)
2301 Metropolis Street
Metropolis, IL 62960-1399
(618) 524-2631

MCDONOUGH (Region 111)
1026 East Jackson Street
Macomb, IL 61455-2520
(309) 833-4127

MCHENRY (Region 11)
2215 Lake Shore Drive
Woodstock, IL 60098-6918
(815) 338-0234

MCLEAN (Region 111)
501 West Washington
PO Box 3725
Bloomington, IL 61702-3725
(309) 451-6000

MENARD (Region IV)
326 East Sangamon
Petersburg, IL 62675-1248
(217) 632-7711

MERCER (Region 111)
400 South East 8th Avenue
Aledo, IL 61231-2095
(309) 582-5178

MONROE (Region V)
123 West Mill Street
PO Box 66
Waterloo, IL 62298-0066
(618) 939-8615

MONTGOMERY (Region IV)
210 East Fairground Avenue
PO Box 515
Hillsboro, IL 62049-0515
(217) 532-3957

MORGAN (Region IV)
45-47 South Central Park Plaza
Jacksonville, IL 62650-2080
(217) 245-5164

MOULTRIE (Region IV)
625 South Hamilton Street
Sullivan, IL 61951-2168
(217) 728-7343

OGLE (Region 11)
2 Pines Plaza
OR, IL 61061-2100
(815) 732-2166

PEORIA (Region 111)
605-607 North East Jefferson Street
Peoria, IL 61603-3899
(309) 671-3282

PERRY (Region V)
314 North Maple Street
DuQuoin, IL 62832-1099
(618) 542-4714

PIATT (Region IV)
108 East Washington Street
PO Box 317
Monticello, IL 61856-0317
(217) 762-9848

PIKE (Region IV)
PO Box 271
Pittsfield, IL 62363-0271
(217) 285-2171

POPE (Region V)
106 North Market Street
PO Box 130
Golconda, IL 62938-0130
(618) 683-2921

PULASKI (Region V)
120 North Front Street
Mounds, IL 62964-1094
(618) 745-9411

PUTNAM (Region 111)
108 South McCoy
PO Box 330
Granville, IL 61326-0330
(815) 339-2164

RANDOLPH (Region V)
870 Lehman Drive
Chester, IL 62233
(618) 826-4559, (617) 826-4558

RICHLAND (Region V)
1406 Martin Street
Olney, IL 62450-4722
(618) 392-3151, (618) 393-7831

ROCK ISLAND (Region 111)
2821 Fifth Street
Rock Island, IL 61201-4085
(309) 794-9530

SALINE (Region V)
320 East Raymond Street
PO Box 724
Harrisburg, IL 62946-0724
(618) 253-7161

SANGAMON (Region IV)
100 South Martin Luther King Drive
Springfield, IL 62703-1197
(217) 782-0400

SCHUYLER (Region IV)
Ill East Washington Street
PO Box 349
Rushville, IL 62681-0349
(217) 322-3377

SCOTT (Region IV)
335 West Cherry Street
Winchester, IL 62694-1029
(217) 742-3158, (217) 742-3159

SHELBY (Region IV)
610 West Main Street
Shelbyville, IL 62565-1440
(217) 774-3971

STARK (Region 111)
213 West Main
PO Box 326
Toulon, IL 61483
(309) 286-2021, (309) 286-7221

STREET CLAIRE/STREET LOUIS (Region V)
225 North 9th Street
East Street Louis, IL 62201-1708
(618) 583-2300

STREET CLAIR/BELLEVILLE (Region V)
1220 Centreville Avenue
Belleville, IL 62220-3007
(618) 257-7400

STEPHENSON (Region 11)
1631 South Galena Avenue
Freeport, IL 61032-2500
(815) 232-6123, (815) 232-6124, (815) 232-6122, (815) 232-6121

TAZEWELL (Region 111)
200 South Second Street, Suite 20
Pekin, IL 61554-4083
(309) 347-4184

UNION (Region V)
201 East Chestnut Street
Anna, IL 62906-1899
(618) 833-2118

VERMILION (Region 111)
220 South Bowman Avenue
PO Box 690
Danville, IL 61834-0690
(217) 442-4003

WABASH (Region V)
229 West 2nd Street
Mt. Carmel, IL 62863-1608
(618) 262-5179, (618) 262-5170, (618) 263-4013

WARREN (Region 111)
1245 South Main Street
PO Box 80
Monmouth, IL 61462-0080
(309) 734-2159

WASHINGTON (Region V)
450 North Kaskaskia
PO Box 72
Nashville, IL 62263
(618) 327-8414, (618) 327-8713

WAYNE (Region V)
215 South East 3rd Street, 2nd Floor
PO Box 207
Fairfield, IL 62837-0207
(618) 842-2621, (618) 842-2622, (618) 842-3431

WHITE (Region V)
1124 West Oak Street
PO Box 639
Carmi, IL 62821-0639
(618) 382-4685

WHITESIDE (Region 11)
2605 Woodlawn Road
Sterling, IL 61081-4151
(815) 632-4045

WILL (Region 11)
45 East Webster Street
Joliet, IL 60432-4067
(815) 740-5350

WILLIAMSON (**Region V**)
1107 West DeYoung, Suite 20
Marion, IL 62959-4403
(618) 997-6591

WINNEBAGO (**Region 11**)
1111 North Avon Street
Rockford, IL 61101-5898
(815) 997-6591

WOODFORD (**Region III**)
107B North Major Street
Eureka, IL 61530-1293
(309) 467-2358

ILLINOIS–LOCAL OFFICE DIRECTORY
(Metro Chicago Offices)

ASHLAND (**Region 1**)
100 North Western Avenue, 2nd Floor
207 Chicago, IL 60612-2222
(312) 633-3700

AUBURN PARK (**Region 1**)
839 West 79th Street
Chicago, IL 60620-2593
(723) 723-8750

AUSTIN (**Region 1**)
408 North Laramie Avenue
Chicago, IL 60644-1999
(773) 854-6300

CALUMET PARK (Region 1)
831 West 119th Street
Chicago, IL 60643-5299
(773) 660-4700

ENGLEWOOD (Region 1)
6305-11 South Western Avenue
Chicago, IL 60636-2495
(773) 918-6700

GARFIELD (Region 1)
500 North Pulaski Road
Chicago, IL 60624-1091
(773) 265-7740

HOSPITAL ASSISTANCE (Region I)
2036 South Michigan, 7' Floor
Chicago, IL 60616-1707
(312) 793-8225

HUMBOLDT PARK (Region 1)
2753 West North Avenue
Chicago, IL 60647-5246
(773) 292-7200

KENWOOD (Region 1)
300 West Pershing Road
Chicago, IL 60609-2822
(773) 538-8000

LOWER NORTH (Region 1)
412 North Milwaukee Avenue
Chicago, IL 60610-3993
(312) 738-5700

MICHIGAN (Region 1)
70 East 21st Street
Chicago, IL 60616-1782
(312) 793-7500

MID-SOUTH (Region I)
(Co-Location Office)
715 East 47th Street, "1" Floor
Chicago, IL 60653
(773) 538-9811 Ext. 333

NORTH ERN (Region 1)
5822 North Western Avenue
Chicago, IL 60659-5097
(773) 989-3600

NORTH WEST (Region 1)
4105 West Chicago Avenue
Chicago, IL 60651-3698
(773) 265-7100

NURSING HOME SERVICES (Region 1)
2036 South Michigan, 6th Floor
Chicago, IL 60616-1793
(312) 793-8000

OAKLAND (Region 1)
610 West Root Street
Chicago, IL 60609-2669
(773) 579-4200

PARK MANOR (Region 1)
724 West 64th Street
Chicago, IL 60621-2792
(773) 602-4700

PERSHING (Region 1)
300 West Pershing Road
Chicago, IL 60609-2896
(773) 538-8900

ROSELAND (Region 1)
11203 South Ellis Avenue
Chicago, IL 60628-4696
(773) 660-7000

SOUTH SUBURBAN (Region 1)
14820 South Kedzie Avenue
Midlothian, IL 60445-3696
(708) 371-5750

SOUTHEAST (Region 1)
8001 South Cottage Grove
Chicago, IL 60619-4095
(773) 602-4200

SPECIAL UNITS (Region 1)
2036 South Michigan, 2nd Floor
Chicago, IL 60616-1793
(312) 793-2740

UPTOWN (Region 1)
2112 West Lawrence Avenue
Chicago, IL 60625-1498
(773) 907-4100

WESTERN (Region 1)
3910 West Ogden
Chicago, IL 60623-2495
(773) 522-8370

WEST SUBURBAN (Region 1)
2701 West Lake
Melrose Park, IL 60160-3041
(708) 338-7600

WICKER PARK (Region 1)
1279 North Milwaukee, 3rd Floor
Chicago, IL 60622-2296
(773) 292-2900

WOODLAWN (Region 1)
915 East 63rd Street
Chicago, IL 60637-3609
(773) 753-5200

ILLINOIS REGIONAL OFFICE DIRECTORY

Division of Community Operations
IL Department of Human Services

Regional Office

DCO Region I-
Cook County South
401 South Clinton, 3rd Floor
Chicago, IL 60607
(312) 793-4131

DCO Region I-
Cook County North and West
401 South Clinton, 3rd Floor
Chicago, IL 60607
(312) 793-4131

DCO Region II
1111 1/4 North Avon Street
Rockford, IL 61101
(815) 987-7826

DCO Region III
1115BN North Street
Peoria, IL 61606
(309) 671-4966

DCO Region IV
208 West Cook
Springfield, IL 62704
(217) 524-6321

DCO Region V
102 East De Young
Marion, IL 62959-2958
(618) 997-2388

INDIANA DIVISION OF FAMILY AND CHILDREN

COUNTY OFFICES

ADAMS
1145 Bollman Street
PO Box 227
Decatur, IN 46733
(219) 724-9169

ALLEN
201 East Rudisill Blvd, Suite 100
Fort Wayne, IN 46806
(219) 458-6200

BARTHOLOMEW
2330 Midway Street, Suite 3
PO Box 587
Columbus, IN 47202-0587
(812) 376-9361

BENTON
403 West 5th Street, Suite B
PO Box 226
Fowler, IN 47944
(765) 884-0120

BLACKFORD
124 North Jefferson Street
PO Box 717
Hartford City, IN 47348
(765) 348-2902

BOONE
953 Monument Drive
PO Box 548
Lebanon, IN 46052
(765) 482-3023

BROWN
121 Locust Lane
PO Box 325
Nashville, IN 47448
(812) 988-2239

CARROLL
U.S. Highway 421 North West
PO Box 276
Delphi, IN 46923-0276
(317) 564-2409

CASS
1714 Dividend Drive
Logansport, IN 46947
(219) 722-3677

CLARK
1200 Madison Street
Clarksville, IN 47129
(812) 288-5400

CLAY
1015 East National Avenue
PO Box 433
Brazil, IN 47834
(812) 448-8731

CLINTON
57 North Jackson Street
PO Box 725
Frankfort, IN 46041
(765) 654-8571

CRAWFORD
304 Indiana Avenue
PO Box 129
English, IN 47118
(812) 338-2701

DAVIESS
4 North East 21st Street
PO Box 618
Washington, IN 47501
(812) 254-0690

DEARBORN
Durban Plaza, 138 Front Street
Lawrenceburg, IN 45725
(812) 537-5131

DECATUR
1025 East Freeland Road, Suite B
Greensburg, IN 47240
(812) 663-6768

DEKALB
934 West 15th Street
PO Box 870
Auburn, IN 46706
(219) 925-2810

DELAWARE
333 South Madison
PO Box 1528
Muncie, IN 47308
(765) 747-7750

DUBOIS
611 Bartley Street
PO Box 230
Jasper, IN 47547
(812) 482-2585

ELKHART
608 Oakland Avenue
Elkhart, IN 46516
(219) 293-6551

FAYETTE
1720 Western Avenue
Connersville, IN 47331
(317) 825-5261

FLOYD
824 University Woods, Suite 9
New Albany, IN 47150
(812) 948-5480

FOUNTAIN
981 East State Street
Veedersburg, IN 47987
(765) 793-4821

FRANKLIN
9127 Oxford Pike, Suite A
Brookville, IN 47012
(765) 647-4081

FULTON
1920 Rhodes Street
Rochester, IN 46975
(219) 223-3413

GIBSON
321South 5th Avenue
Princeton, IN 47670
(812) 385-4727

GRANT
840 North Miller Avenue
Marion, IN 46952
(765) 668-4500

GREENE
Highway 231 South
PO Box 443
Bloomfield, IN 47424
(812) 384-4404

HAMILTON
938 North Tenth Street
Noblesville, IN 46060
(317) 773-2183

HANCOCK
120 West Mckenzie, Suite F
Greenfield, IN 46140
(317) 467-6360

HARRISON
2026 Highway 337 North West
PO Box 366
Corydon, IN 47112
(812) 738-8166

HENDRICKS
6781 East US 36, Suite 200
Danville, IN 47122
(317) 272-4917

HENRY
1416 Broad Street, 2nd Floor
New Castle, IN 47362
(765) 529-3450

HOWARD
105 West Sycamore Street
Kokomo, IN 46901
(765) 457-9410

HUNTINGTON
88 Home Street
Huntington, IN 46750
(219) 356-4420

JACKSON
220 South Main Street
PO Box C
Brownstown, IN 47220
(812) 358-2421

JASPER
215 West Kellner Blvd, Suite 16
PO Box 279
Rensselaer, IN 47978
(219) 866-4186

JAY
7959 Highway 67 West
PO Box 1034
Portland, IN 47371
(219) 726-7933

JEFFERSON
1405 Bear Street
Madison, IN 47250
(812) 265-2027

JENNINGS
939 Veterans Drive
PO Box 905
North Vernon, IN 47265
(812) 346-2254

JOHNSON
80 South Jackon Street
Franklin, IN 46131
(317) 736-3730

KNOX
1050 Washington Avenue
PO Box 235
Vincennes, IN 47591
(812) 882-3920

KOSCIUSKO
205 North Lake Street
Warsaw, IN 46580
(219) 267-8108

LAGRANGE
421-B South Detroit Street
Lagrange, IN 46761
(219) 463-3451

LAKE
839 Broadway
Gary, IN 46402
(219) 881-2037
(219) 881-2020

LAPORTE
1230 State Road 2 West
PO Box 1402
LaPorte, IN 46352
(219) 326-5870

LAWRENCE
918 16th Street, Suite 100
Bedford, IN 47421-3824
(812) 279-9706

MADISON
222 East 10th Street
Suite D
Anderson, IN 46016
(765) 649-0142

MARION
129 East Market Street
Indianapolis, IN 46204
Please refer to offices listed
throughout Marion Co.

MARSHALL
1850 Walter Glaub Drive
PO Box 539
Plymouth, IN 46563
(219) 935-4046

MARTIN
51 Ravine Street Box 88
Shoals, IN 47581
(812) 247-2871

MIAMI
1250 West Main
PO Box 143
Peru, IN 46970-0143
(765) 473-6611

MONROE
401 East Miller Drive
Bloomington, IN 47401
(812) 336-6351

MONTGOMERY
307 Binford Street
Crawfordsville, IN 47933
(765) 362-5600

MORGAN
1250 South Morton Avenue
Martinsville, IN 46151
(765) 342-7101

NEWTON
250 East State Street
PO Box 520
Morocco, IN 47963
(219) 285-2206

NOBLE
107 Weber Road
Albion, IN 46701
(219) 636-2021

OHIO
125 North Walnut
PO Box 196
Rising Sun, IN 47040
(812) 438-2530

ORANGE
326 North Gospel, PO Box 389
Paoli, IN 47454
(812) 723-3616

OWEN
14 North Washington Street
Spencer, IN 47460
(812) 829-2281

PARKE
116 West Ohio
Rockville, IN 47872
(765) 569-3156

PERRY
316 East Highway 66
Tell City, IN 47586
(812) 547-7055

PIKE
2105 East Main
Petersburg, IN 47567
(812) 354-9716

PORTER
152 Indiana Avenue
Valparaiso, IN 46383
(219) 462-2112

POSEY
1809 Main Street
PO Box 568
Mount Vernon, IN 47620
(812) 838-4429

PULASKI
614 West 11th Street, PO Box 130
Winamac, IN 46996
(219) 946-3312

PUTNAM
620 Tennessee Street, Suite 1
Greencastle, IN 46135
(765) 653-9780

RANDOLPH
2 Omco Square, Suite 200
Winchester, IN 47394
(765) 584-2811

RIPLEY
630 South Adams, PO Box 215
Versailles, IN 47042
(812) 689-6295

RUSH
1340 North Cherry
Rushville, IN 46173
(765) 932-2392

STREET JOSEPH
701 South Chapin Street, PO Box 4638
South Bend, IN 46634
(219) 236-5300

SCOTT
705 West Fairground Road
PO Box 424
Scottsburg, IN 47170
(812) 752-2503

SHELBY
42 East Washington Street
PO Box 849
Shelbyville, IN 46176
(317) 392-5040

SPENCER
900 Old Plank Road
Rockport, IN 47635
(812) 649-9111

STARKE
318 East Culver Road
Knox, IN 46534
(219) 722-3411

STEUBEN
317 South Wayne Street, Suite 2a
Angola, IN 46703
(219) 665-3713

SULLIVAN
128 South State Street
Sullivan, IN 47882
(812) 268-6326

SWITZERLAND
801 East Main Street, PO Box 98
Vevay, IN 47043
(812) 426-3232

TIPPECANOE
324 South Street
Lafayette, IN 47901-1304
(765) 742-0400

TIPTON
Courthouse-Box 36
Tipton, IN 46072
(765) 675-7441

UNION
303A North Main Street
PO Box 344
Liberty, IN 47353
(765) 458-5121

VANDERBURGH
100 East Sycamore Street
PO Box 154
Evansville, IN 47701-0154
(812) 421-5500

VERMILLION
215 West Extension Street
PO Box 218
Newport, IN 47966
(765) 492-3305

VIGO
30 North 8th Street
Terre Haute, IN 47807
(812) 234-0100

WABASH
89 West Canal Street
Wabash, IN 46992
(219) 563-8471

WARREN
5 Railroad Street
Williamsport, IN 47993
(765) 762-6125

WARRICK
1302 Millis Avenue
PO Box 265
Boonville, IN 47601
(812) 897-2270

WASHINGTON
12 Westminster Center
Salem, IN 47167
(812) 883-4305

WAYNE
25 South Second
Richmond, IN 47374
(765) 935-0078

WELLS
114 South Main Place
PO Box 495
Bluffton, IN 46714
(219) 824-3530

WHITE
715 North Main Street
PO Box 365
Monticello, IN 47960
(219) 583-5742

WHITLEY
115 South Line Street
Columbia City, IN 46725
(219) 244-6331

IOWA DEPARTMENT OF HUMAN SERVICES

ADAIR
132 South East Court Drive
Greenfield, IA 50849
(515) 743-2119

ADAMS
Courthouse
Corning, IA 50841
(515) 322-4031

ALLAMAKEE
Courthouse
Waukon, IA 52172
(319) 568-4583

APPANOOSE
209 East Jackson Street
Centerville, IA 52544
(515) 437-4450

AUDUBON
210 North Market Street
audubon, IA 50025-1255
(712) 563-4259

BENTON
114 East Fourth Street
Vinton, IA 52349
(319) 472-4746

BLACK HAWK
1407 Independence Avenue
Waterloo, IA 50704-7500
(319) 291-2441

BOONE
900 West Mamie Eisenhower
Boone, IA 50036
(515) 433-0593

BREMER
209-20th Street North West
Waverly, IA 50677
(319) 352-4233

BUCHANAN
1413 First Street
West Independence, IA 50644
(319) 334-6091

BUENA VISTA
311 East Fifth Street
Storm Lake, IA 50588
(712) 749-2536

BUTLER
315 North Main
Allsion, IA 50602
(319) 267-2594

CALHOUN
515 Court Street
Rockweell City, IA 50579
(712) 297-8524

CARROLL
515 North Main Street
Carroll, IA 51401-2346
(712) 792-4391

CASS
Courthouse
Atlantic, IA 50022
(712) 243-4401

CEDAR
101 Lynn Street
Tipton, IA 52772
(319) 886-6036

CERRO GORDO
Mohawk Square
22 North Georgia Avenue
Mason City, IA 50401
(515) 424-8641

CHEROKEE
239 West Maple Street
Cherokee, IA 51012
(712) 225-6723

CHICKASAW
910 East Main Street
New Hampton, IA 50659
(515) 394-4315

CLARKE
115 North Main Street
Osceola, IA 50213
(515) 342-6516

CLAY
217 West Fifth Street
Spencer, IA 51301
(712) 262-3586

CLAYTON
Clayton County Office Building
100 Sandpit Road
Elkader, IA 52043
(319) 245-1766

CLINTON
121 Sixth Avenue South
Clinton, IA 52732
(319) 242-0573

CRAWFORD
107 South Main Street
Denison, IA 51442
(712) 263-5668

DALLAS
210 North 10th Street
Adel, IA 50003
(515) 993-5817

DAVIS
203 South Madison Street
Bloomfield, IA 52537
(515) 664-2239

DECATUR
210 North Main Street
Leon, IA 50144
(515) 446-4312

DELAWARE
721 South Fifth Street
Manchester, IA 52057
(319) 927-4512

DES MOINES
409 North Fourth Street
Burlington, IA 52601
(319) 754-4622

DICKINSON
901-20th Street
Spirit Lake, IA 51360
(712) 336-2555

DUBUQUE
Town Clock Plaza
Nesler Center, Suite 410
Dubuque, IA 52001
(319) 557-8251

EMMET
220 South First Street
Estherville, IA 51334
(712) 362-7237

FAYETTE
129 A North Vine Street
Union, IA 52175
(319) 422-5634

FLOYD
1206 South Main Street
Charles City, IA 50616
(515) 228-5713

FRANKLIN
19 Second Avenue
Hampton, IA 50441
(515) 456-4763

FREMONT
414 Clay Street
Sidney, IA 51652
(712) 374-2512

GREENE
114 North Chestnut Street
Jefferson, IA 50129-2144
(515) 386-2143

GRUNDY
315 North Main Street
Allison, IA 50602
(319) 267-2594

GUTHRIE
200 North Fifth Avenue
Gutherie Center, IA 50115-1331
(515) 747-2293

HAMILTON
2300 South Superior Street
Webster City, IA 50595
(515) 832-9555

HANCOCK
120 East Eighth Street
Garner, IA 50438
(515) 923-3758

HARDIN
1201-14th Avenue
Eldora, IA 50627
(515) 939-8141

HARRISON
204 East Sixth Street
Logan, IA 51546
(712) 644-2460

HENRY
205 West Madison
Mount Pleasant, IA 52641
(319) 986-5157

HOWARD
205 East Second Street
Cresco, IA 52136
(319) 547-2860

HUMBOLDT
Courthouse
Dakota City, IA 50529
(515) 332-3383

IDA
Courthouse
Ida Grove, IA 51445
(712) 364-2631

IOWA
1061 Court Avenue
Marengo, IA 51445
(712) 642-5573

JACKSON
700 West Quarry
Maquoketa, IA 52060
(319) 652-4000

JASPER
120 First Street North , Suite 500
Newton, IA 50208
(515) 792-1955

JEFFERSON
51 West Hempstead Street
Fairfield, IA 52556
(515) 471-2011

JOHNSON
911 North Governor Street
Iowa City, IA 52240
(319) 356-6050

JONES
500 West Main Street
Anamosa, IA 52205
(319) 462-3557

KEOKUK
Route 1
Sigourney, IA52591
(515) 622-2090

KOSSUTH
109 West State Street
Algona, IA 50511
(515) 295-7771

LEE (NORTH)
933 Avenue H
Fort Madison, IA 52627
(319) 372-3651

LEE (SOUTH)
107 Bank Street
Keokuk, IA 52632
(319) 524-1052

LINN
411 Third Street, South East
Suite 400
Cedar Rapids, IA 52401
(319) 398-3950

LOUISA
317 Van Buren Street
Wapello, IA 52653
(319) 523-6351

LUCAS
125 South Grand Street
Chariton, IA 50049
(515) 774-5071

LYON
803 South Greene Street, Suite 2
Rock Rapids, IA 51246
(712) 472-3743

MADISON
209 East Madison Street
Winterset, IA 50273
(515) 462-2931

MAHASKA
Heartland Square Mall
410 South 11th Street
Oskaloosa, IA 52577
(515) 673-3496

MARION
Old Highway 92 East
Knoxville, IA 50138
(515) 842-5087

MARSHALL
206 West State Street
Marshalltown, IA 50158
(515) 752-6741

MILLS
711 South Vine Street
Glenwood, IA 51534
(712) 527-4803

MITCHELL
1206 South Main Street
Charles City, IA 50616
(515) 228-5713

MONONA
610 Iowa Avenue
Onawa, IA 51040
(712) 423-1921

MONROE
103 South Clinton
Albia, IA 52531
(515) 932-5187

MONTGOMERY
1109 Highland Avenue
Red Oak, IA 51566
(712) 623-4838

MUSCATINE
120 East Third Street, 4th Floor
Muscatine, IA 52761
(319) 263-9302

O'BRIEN
160 Second Street, South East
Primghar, IA 51245
(712) 757-5135

OSCEOLA
110 Cedar Lane
Sibley, IA 51249
(712) 754-3622

PAGE
121 South 15th Street, Suite C
Clarinda, IA 51632
(712) 542-5111

PALO ALTO
2105 Main Street
Emmetsburg, IA 50536
(712) 852-2832

PLYMOUTH
19 Second Avenue, North West
LeMars, IA 51031
(712) 546-8877

POCAHONTAS
23 Third Avenue, North East
Pocahontas, IA 50574
(712) 335-3565

POLK
City View Plaza
1200 University Avenue
Des Moines, IA 50314-2330
(515) 283-7900

POLK (CENTRAL OFFICE)
1900 Carpenter
Des Moines, IA 50314-1309
(515) 286-3555

POLK (EAST OFFICE)
1740 Garfield
Des Moines, IA 50316-2646
(515) 286-3270

POLK (PIONEER COLUMBUS OFFICE)
2100 South East Fifth
Des Moines, IA 50315-1552
(515) 288-9333

POTTAWATTAMIE
417 East Kanesville Boulevard
Council Bluffs, IA 51503
(712) 328-5648

POWESHIEK
718 Industrial Avenue
Grinnell, IA 50112
(515) 236-3149

RINGGOLD
Courthouse
Mount Ayr, IA 50854
(515) 464-2247

SAC
116 South State Street
Sac City, IA 50583
(712) 662-4782

SCOTT
428 Western Avenue, 2nd Floor
Davenport, IA 52801
(319) 326-8680

SHELBY
807 Court Street
Harlan, IA 51537
(712) 755-3145

SIOUX
215 Central Avenue, South East
Orange City, IA 51041
(712) 737-2943

STORY
126 South Kellogg
Ames, IA 50014
(515) 292-2035

TAMA
129 West High Street
Toledo, IA 52342
(515) 484-3406

TAYLOR
309 Main Street
Bedford, IA 50833
(712) 523-2129

UNION
Courthouse
Creston, IA 50801
(515) 782-2173

VAN BUREN
Courthouse
Keosauqua, IA 52565
(319) 293-3791

WAPELLO
120 East Main Street
Ottumwa, IA 52501
(515) 682-8793

WARREN
901 East Iowa Street
Indianola, IA 50125
(515) 961-5353

WASHINGTON
108 West Jefferson Street
Washington, IA 52353
(319) 653-7752

WAYNE
117 West Jackson Street
Corydon, IA 50060
(515) 872-1820

WEBSTER
330 First Avenue, North
Dodge, IA 50501
(515) 955-6353

WINNEBAGO
216 South Clark Street
Forest City, IA 50436
(515) 582-3271

WINNESHIEK
305 Montgomery Street
Decorah, IA 52101
(319) 382-2928

WOODBURY
822 Douglas Street
Sioux City, IA 51101-1122
(712) 255-0833

WORTH
22 North Georgia Avenue
Mason City, IA 50401
(515) 424-8641

WRIGHT
114 First Street, South West
Clarion, IA 50525
(515) 532-6645

KANSAS AREA CONTACTS

CHANUTE
1500 West 7th.
Chanute, KS 66720
(316) 431-5000
Counties Served:
Allen, Anderson, Bourbon, Cherokee, Crawford, Labette, Linn, Montgomery, Neosho, Wilson, Woodson

EMPORIA
1015 Scott
Emporia, KS 66801
(316) 342-2505
Counties Served:
Butler, Chase, Chautauqua, Coffey, Cowley, Elk, Greenwood, Lyon, Marion, Morris, Osage

GARDEN CITY
1710 Palace Drive
Garden City, KS 67846
(316) 272-5800
Counties Served:
Barber, Clark, Comanche, Edwards, Finney, Ford, Grant, Gray, Greeley, Hamilton, Haskell, Hodgeman, Kearney, Kiowa, Lane, Meade, Morton, Ness,Pratt, Scott, Seward, Stafford, Stanton, Stevens, Wichita

HAYS
1105 East 30th
Hays, KS 67601
(785) 628-1066
Counties Served:
Barton, Cheyenne, Decatur, Ellis, Grove, Graham, Logan, Norton, Osborne, Pawnee, Phillips, Rawlins, Rooks, Rush, Russell, Sheridan, Sherman, Smith, Thomas, Trego, Wallace

HUTCHINSON
600 Andrew South
Hutchinson, KS 67505
(316) 663-5731
Counties Served:
Harper, Harvey, Kingman, McPerson, Reno, Rice, Summer

KANSAS CITY
400 State Avenue
Kansas City, KS 66101
(913) 279-7000
Counties Served:
Wyandotte

LAWRENCE
PO Box 590, Lawrence KS 66044-0590 (mailing address)
1901 Delaware
Lawrence, KS 66046 (physical address)
(785) 832-3700
Counties Served:
Atchinson, Brown, Doniphan, Douglas, Franklin, Jackson, Jefferson

MANHATTAN
2709 Amherst
Manhattan, KS 66502
(785) 776-4011
Counties Served:
Clay, Cloud, Dickinson, Ellsworth, Geary, Jewell, Lincoln, Marshall, Mitchell, Nemaha, Ottawa, Pottawatomie, Republic, Riley, Salina, Wabaunsee, Washington

OLATHE
401 West Frontier Lane
Olathe, KS 66001
(913) 768-3300
Counties Served:
Johnson, Leavenuenworth, Miami

TOPEKA
235 South Kansas
Topeka, KS 66603
(785) 296-2500
Counties Served:
Shawnee

WICHITA
230 East William
Wichita, KS 67202
(316) 337-7000
Counties Served:
Sedgwick

KENTUCKY

BARREN RIVER REGION-COUNTIES:
Allen, Barren, Butler, Edmonson, Hart, Logan, Metcalfe, Monroe,
Simpson, Warren

ALLEN
505 East Main Street
Scottsville, KY 42164
270-237-3661
Fax: (270) 237-5365

BARREN
734 East Main Street
PO Box 218
Glasgow, KY 42142-0218
(270) 651-5119
Fax: (270) 651-6465

BUTLER
201 West Ohio Street
PO Box 627
Morgantown, KY 42261-0627
(270) 526-3395
Fax: (270) 526-6776

EDMONSON
Highway 259 South
PO Box 539
Brownsville, KY 42210-0539
(270) 597-2118
Fax: (270) 597-2788

HART
810 National Turnpike
PO Box 489
Munfordville, KY 42765-0489
(270) 524-7211
Fax: (270) 524-2556

LOGAN
345 West Third Street
Russellville, KY 42276
(270) 726-9557
Fax: (270) 725-9475

MEDCALFE
Tompkinsville Road
PO Box 357
Edmonton, KY 42129
(270) 432-2521
Fax: (270) 432-2722

MONROE
201 West Paige Street
PO Box 578
Tompkinsville, KY 42167-0578
(270) 487-6798
Fax: (270) 487-8138

SIMPSON
210 West Cedar Street
Franklin, KY 42134
(270) 586-4433
Fax: (270) 586-6495

WARREN
1010 State Street, Suite 2
PO Box 1929
Bowling Green, KY 42102-1929
(270) 746-7850
Fax: (270) 746-7035

BIG SANDY REGION-COUNTIES:

Floyd, Johnson, Magoffin, Martin, Pike

FLOYD
895 North Lake Drive
Prestonsburg, KY 41653
(606) 886-3871
Fax: (606) 889-9063

JOHNSON
Coleman Bldg
11th Street & Stafford Avenue
PO Box 1424
Paintsville, KY 41240
(606) 789-5307
Fax: (606) 789-5952

MAGOFFIN
125 South Church Street
PO Box 89
Salyersville, KY 41465
606-349-6131
Fax: (606) 349-6033

MARTIN
Main Street
PO Box 408
Inez, KY 41224
(606) 298-3577
Fax: (606) 298-0311

PIKE
1300 Hambley Blvd
PO Box 3249
Pikeville, KY 41501
(606) 433-7760
Fax: (606) 433-7100

BLUEGRASS (FAYETTE) REGION-COUNTIES:

FAYETTE
1350 East New Circle Road
Lexington, KY 40505
(606) 246-2070
Fax: (606) 246-2515

BLUEGRASS (RURAL) REGION-COUNTIES:
Anderson, Bouron, Boyle, Clark, Estill, Franklin, Garrard, Harrison, Jessamine, Lincoln, Madison, Mercer, Nicholas, Powell, Scott, Woodford

ANDERSON
329 Court Street
Lawrenceburg, KY 40342
(502) 839-6933
Fax: (502) 839-5712

BOURBON
Paris Municipal Building
525 High Street, 2nd Floor
PO Box 139
Paris, KY 40361
(606) 987-2455
Fax: (606) 987-9041

BOYLE
1000 East Lexington Avenue
Suite 6
Danville, KY 40422
(606) 239-7837
Fax: (606) 239-7010

CLARK
11 South Highland Street
PO Box 75
Winchester, KY 40392-0075
(606) 737-7730
Fax: (606) 737-7549

ESTILL
102 Mack Street
PO Box 506
Irvine, KY 40336
(606) 723-5124
Fax: (606) 723-2915

FRANKLIN
102 Mero Street
Frankfort, KY 40601
(502) 564-6636
Fax: (502) 564-9751

GARRARD
124 Pleasant Retreat Plaza
Lancaster, KY 40444
(606) 792-2701
Fax: (606) 792-2701

HARRISON
Rt 7, PO Box 47
Cynthiana KY 41031
(606) 234-4151
Fax: (606) 234-3465

JESSAMINE
111 Edgewood Plaza
Nicholasville, KY 40356
(606) 885-3361
Fax: (606) 887-9350

LINCOLN
1710 US 27 North
PO Box 385
Stanford, KY 40484
(606) 365-2171
Fax: (606) 365-8285

MADISON
126 South Killarney Lane
PO Box 240
Richmond, KY 40476-0240
(606) 623-1310
Fax: (606) 626-3112

MERCER
661 Beaumont Plaza Street
PO Box 386
Harrodsburg, KY 40330-0486
(606) 734-7724
Fax: (606) 734-0856

NICHOLAS
226 Locust Street
PO Box 335
Carlisle, KY 40311
(606) 289-7101
Fax: (606) 389-4535

POWELL
124 North Main Street
PO Box 550
Stanton, KY 40380
(606) 663-2293
Fax: (606) 663-9399

SCOTT
1000 West Main Street
Suite #2
Georgetown, KY 40324
(502) 863-1381
Fax: (502) 863-1069

WOODFORD
125 Lexington Street
Versailles, KY 40383
(606) 873-3191
Fax: (606) 873-8410

CUMBERLAND VALLEY REGION-COUNTIES:
Bell, Clay, Harlan, Jackson, Knox, Laurel, Rockcastle, Whitley

BELL
124 Kentucky Avenue
PO Drawer 189
Pineville, KY 40977
(606) 337-7055
Fax: (606) 337-9967

CLAY
Hatcher Building
Rt. #3
PO Box 409
Manchester, KY 40962
(606) 598-2118
Fax: (606) 598-0569

HARLAN
115 South Cumberland Avenue
PO Box 939
Harlan, KY 40831
(606) 573-2120
Fax: (606) 573-4789

JACKSON
Vickers Building
US Highway 421 Box 248
McKee, KY 40447
(606) 287-7131
Fax: (606) 387-4113

KNOX
209 Knox Street
PO Box 610
Barbourville, KY 40906
(606) 546-3121
Fax: (606) 545-9104

LAUREL
31 South Laurel Road
London, KY 40744
(606) 864-6811
Fax: (606) 877-9018

ROCKCASTLE
Jct. 25-Highway 150
PO Box 1019
Mt. Vernon, KY 40456
(606) 256-2481
Fax: (606) 256-3475

WHITLEY
408 East Center Street
Corbin, KY 40701
(606) 528-5745
Fax: (606) 528-2417

FIVCO REGION-COUNTIES:
Boyd, Carter, Elliott, Greenup, Lawrence

BOYD
411 19th Street
PO Box 750
Ashland, KY 41105-0750
(606) 920-2013
Fax: (606) 920-2082

CARTER
211 West Main Street
PO Box 910
Grayson, KY 41143
(606) 474-5103
Fax: (606) 474-2898

ELLIOTT
Weddington Building
HC 81, Box 328
Sandy Hook, KY 41171
(606) 738-5193
Fax: (606) 738-5183

GREENUP
1103 Seaton Avenue
PO Box 707
Greenup, KY 41144
(606) 473-7311
Fax: (606) 473-9126

LAWRENCE
122 Rice Street
PO Box 768
Louisa, KY 41230-0768
(606) 638-4526
Fax: (606) 638-0796

GATEWAY/BUFFALO TRACE REGION-COUNTIES:
Bath, Bracken, Fleming, Lewis, Mason, Menifee, Montgomery, Morgan, Robertson, Rowan

BATH
Miller Building
44 Coyle Street
PO Box 7
Owingsville, KY 40360
(606) 674-6344
Fax: (606) 674-3920

BRACKEN
111 Locust Street
PO Box 235
Brooksville, KY 41004
(606) 735-2193
Fax: (606) 735-3716

FLEMING
101B Clark Street
PO Box 271
Flemingsburg, KY 41041
(606) 845-7561
Fax: (606) 845-9004

LEWIS
317 Second Street
PO Box 39
Vanceburg, KY 41179
(606) 796-3037
Fax: (606) 796-3595

MASON
930 1/2 Forest Avenue
PO Box 196
Maysville, KY 41056-0196
(606) 564-6876
Fax: (606) 564-3612

MENIFEE
Route 36
PO Box 50
Frenchburg, KY 40322
(606) 768-2118
Fax: (606) 768-6118

MONTGOMERY
212 Locust Street
PO Box 219
Mt. Sterling, KY 40353
(606) 498-5398
Fax: (606) 497-0849

MORGAN
324 Glenn Avenue
PO Box 519
West Liberty, KY 41472
(606) 743-3127
Fax: (606) 743-3221

ROBERTSON
Main Street
PO Box 200
Mt. Olivet, KY 41064-0200
(606) 724-5414
Fax: (606) 724-2046

ROWAN
102 West Main Street
PO Box 886
Morehead, KY 40351
(606) 784-6602
Fax: (606) 784-7769

GREEN RIVER REGION-COUNTIES:

Davies, Hancock, Henderson, McLean, Ohio, Union, Webster

DAVIES

311 West Second Street
Owensboro, KY 42301
(270) 687-7278
Fax: (270) 687-7360

HANCOCK

318 Main-Cross Street
PO Box 7
Hawesville, KY 42348
(270) 927-8156
Fax: (270) 927-8775

HENDERSON

228 North Green Street
Henderson, KY 42420
(270) 826-8351
Fax: (270) 820-0112

McLean

255 West Main Street
PO Box 278
Island, KY 42350
(270) 486-3206
Fax: (270) 486-9285

OHIO
927 West 7th Street
PO Box 309
Beaver Dam, KY 42320
(270) 274-8996
Fax: (279) 274-8998

UNION
122 North Court Street
Morganfield, KY 42437
(270) 389-1892
Fax: (270) 389-9255

WEBSTER
26 South Main
PO Box 80
Dixon, KY 42409
(270) 639-5044
Fax: (270) 639-9125

KENTUCKY RIVER REGION-COUNTIES:
Breathitt, Knott, Lee, Leslie, Letcher, Owsley, Perry, Wolfe

BREATHITT
355 Broadway
PO Box 728
Jackson, KY 41339
(606) 666-2481
Fax: (606) 666-9760

KNOTT
Highway 550 West
PO Box 668
Hindman, KY 41822
(606) 785-3137
Fax: (606) 785-5699

LEE
Lee County Courthouse
256 Main Street, Drawer 1
Beattyville, KY 41311
(606) 464-2404
Fax: (606) 464-9909

LESLIE
Hyden Plaza
Highway 421 South
PO Box 930
Hyden, KY 41749
(606) 672-2306
Fax: (606) 672-6991

LETCHER
65A North Webb Street
Whitesburg, KY 41858
(606) 633-9332
Fax: (606) 633-0145

OWSLEY
Main Street
PO Box 308
Booneville, KY 41314
(606) 593-5133
Fax: (606) 593-7526

PERRY
742 High Street
Hazard, KY 41701
(606) 435-6043
Fax: (606) 435-6125

WOLFE
Murphy Building, 1st Floor
330 Main Street
PO Box 9
Campton, KY 41301
(606) 668-3175
Fax: (606)-668-7280

KIPDA (JEFFERSON) REGION-COUNTIES:

JEFFERSON
Valley Neighborhood Place
10200 Dixie Highway
2nd Floor
Louisville, KY 40272
(502) 995-3000
(502) 995-3001
Fax: (502) 995-3010

JEFFERSON
Fairdale Neighborhood Place
1000 Neighborhood Place
Fairdale, KY 40118
(502) 363-1485
Fax: (502) 363-1435

JEFFERSON
3307 Indian Trail
Louisville, KY 40213
(502) 962-5660

JEFFERSON
1st Neighborhood Place-Thomas Jefferson
4401 Rangeland Road
Louisville, KY 40219
(502) 961-6180
Fax: (502) 962-3171 and (502) 595-4634

JEFFERSON
908 West Broadway
L&N Building
Louisville, KY 40203
(502) 595-4014 and (502) 595-4679 and (502) 595-4712
(502) 595-4298 and (502) 595-4971 and (502) 595-4857
(502) 595-4174 and (502) 595-4351 and (502) 595-4872
(502) 595-4319 and (502) 595-4290
Fax: (502) 595-4634 and (502) 595-4722 and (502) 595-4863

JEFFERSON
Cane Run Neighborhood Place
3410 Lees Lane
Louisville, KY 40216
(502) 485-6814
Fax: (502) 485-6818

KIPDA (Rural) Region-Counties:
Bullitt, Henry, Oldham, Shelby, Spencer, Trimble

BULLITT
445 Highway 44 East
Suite 209
Shepherdsville, KY 40165
(502) 543-7081
Fax: (502) 543-3819

HENRY
1427 Campellsburg Road
PO Box 328
New Castle, KY 40050
(502) 845-2110
Fax: (502) 845-1856

OLDHAM
300 North First Street
LaGrange, KY 40031
(502) 222-9191
Fax: (502) 222-5813

SHELBY
17 Village Plaza
U S 60 West
Shelbyville, KY 40065
(502) 633-3530
Fax: (502) 633-0737

SPENCER
73 East Main Street
PO Box 338
Taylorsville, KY 40071
(502) 477-2224
Fax: (502) 477-5679

TRIMBLE
Bedford Professional Building
18 Alexander Avenue
Highway 42 West
PO Box 246
Bedford, KY 40006
(502) 255-3278
Fax: (502) 255-4609

LAKE CUMBERLAND REGION-COUNTIES:
Adair, Casey, Clinton, Cumberland, Green, McCreary, Pulaski, Russell, Taylor, Wayne

ADAIR
703 Jamestown Street
PO Box 429
Columbia, KY 42728-0429
(270) 384-2163
Fax: (270) 384-5875

CASEY
137 Courthouse Square
PO Box 1437
Liberty, KY 42539-1437
(606) 787-8338
Fax: (606) 787-0721

CLINTON
107 East Water Street
Albany, KY 42602
(606) 387-6446
Fax: (606) 387-7254

CUMBERLAND
232 Keen Street
PO Box 397
Burkesville, KY 42717-0397
(270) 864-2556
Fax: (270) 864-4129

GREEN
116 North Main Street
Greensburg, KY 42743
(270) 932-7484
Fax: (270) 932-5051

MCCREARY
Highway 27
Whitley City Plaza
PO Box 457
Whitley City, KY 42653-0457
(606) 376-5304
Fax: (606) 376-9538

PULASKI
650 North Main Street
Suite 250
PO Box 1323
Somerset, KY 42502
(606) 677-4103
Fax: (606) 677-4143

RUSSELL
Bates Building
South Main Street
PO Box 770
Jamestown, KY 42629-0770
(270) 343-3196
Fax: (270) 343-5663

TAYLOR
156 Gaines Drive, Office A
Campbellsville, KY 42718
(270) 565-6621
Fax: (270) 789-4095

WAYNE
Tradeway Shopping Center
PO Box 697
Monticello, KY 42633-0697
(606) 348-3321
Fax: (606) 348-0366

LINCOLN TRAIL REGION-COUNTIES:
Breckinridge, Grayson, Hardin, Larue, Meade, Marion, Nelson, Washington

BRECKINRIDGE
110 US 60 East
PO Box 550
Hardinsburg, KY 40143-0550
(270) 756-2156
Fax: (270) 756-1684

GRAYSON
Southgate Mall
498 South Main Street
PO Box 168
Leitchfield, KY 42755-0168
(270) 259-4041
Fax: (270) 259-0646

HARDIN
916 North Mulberry Street
Elizabethtown, KY 42701
(270) 766-5029
Fax: (270) 766-5163

LARUE
30 Shawnee Drive
Hodgenville, KY 42748-0169
(720) 358-3176
Fax: (270) 358-8569

MARION
118 East Mulberry Street
PO Box 605
Lebanon, KY 40033-0605
(270) 692-6036
Fax: (270) 692-6485

MEADE
516 By-Pass Road
Brandenburg, KY 40108-1702
(270) 422-3974
Fax: (279) 692-6485

NELSON
901 Atkinson Hill Avenue
PO Box 306
Bardstown, KY 40004-0306
(502) 348-9282
Fax: (502) 349-6450

WASHINGTON
108 Progress Street
PO Box 407
Springfield, KY 40069
(606) 336-3977
Fax: (606) 336-0034

NORTH ERN KENTUCKY REGION-COUNTIES:

Boone, Campbell, Carroll, Gallatin, Grant, Kenton, Owen, Pendleton

BOONE
Suite 105
7711 Ewing Boulevard
Florence, KY 41042
(606) 371-6900
Fax: (606) 371-5103

CAMPBELL
Watertower Square
Suite 4
601 Washington Avenue
Newport, KY 41071
(606) 292-6707
Fax: (606) 292-6427

CARROLL
216 5th Street
PO Box 368
Carrollton, KY 41008
(502) 732-4271
Fax: (502) 732-8708

GALLATIN
300-A Main-Cross Street
PO Box 555
Warsaw, KY 41095
(606) 567-7281
Fax: (606) 567-2341

GRANT
120 North Main Street
Williamstown, KY 41097
(606) 824-5202
Fax: (606) 824-7910

KENTON
20 East Seventh Steet, 3rd Floor
Covington, KY 41011
(606) 292-6600
Fax: (606) 292-6365

OWEN
110 North Madison Street
PO Box 445
Owenton, KY 40359
(502) 484-3458
Fax: (502) 484-0698

PENDLETON
510 Wilson Street
Falmouth, KY 41040
(606) 654-6123
Fax: (606) 654-5868

PENNYRILE REGION-COUNTIES:
Caldwell, Christian, Crittenden, Hopkins, Livingston, Lyon, Muhlenberg, Todd, Trigg

CALDWELL
102 South Seminary Street
PO Box 646
Princeton, KY 42445-0646
(270) 365-5524
Fax: (270) 365-6763

CHRISTIAN
Brickyard Plaza
644 North Drive
PO Box 524
Hopkinsville, KY 42241-0524
(270) 889-6512
Fax: (270) 889-6027

CRITTENDEN
135 East Carlisle Street
PO Box 435
Marion, KY 42064-0435
(270) 965-2254
Fax: (270) 965-2424

HOPKINS
1086 Thornberry Drive
Madisonville, KY 42431
(270) 824-7555
Fax: (279) 824-7588

LIVINGSTON
104 West Adair Street
PO Box 227
Smithland, KY 42081-0227
(270) 928-2102
Fax: (270) 928-3120

LYON
656 Trade Avenue
PO Box 557
Eddyville, KY 42038-0557
(270) 388-2206
Fax: (270) 388-0852

MUHLENBERG
518 Hopkinsville Street
PO Box 369
Greenville, KY 42345-0369
(270) 338-2330
Fax: (270) 338-4311

TODD
102 North Williams Lane
PO Box 279
Elkton, KY 42220-0279
(279) 265-2596
Fax: (270) 265-4283

TRIGG
28 Main Street
PO Box 644
Cadiz, KY 42211-0644
(270) 522-6671
Fax: (270) 522-4283

PURCHASE REGION-COUNTIES:
Ballard, Calloway, CArlisle, Fulton, GrAvenues, Hickman, McCracken, Marshall

BALLARD
323 Broadway
PO Box 389
LaCenter, KY 42056-0389
(270) 665-5158
Fax: (270) 665-9450

CALLOWAY
203 South 6th Street
PO Box 865
Murray, KY 42071-0865
(270) 753-1871
Fax: (270) 753-1817

CARLISLE
140 Front Street
PO Box 368
Bardwell, KY 42023-0368
(270) 628-5442
Fax: (279) 628-0161

FULTON
320 Mears Street
PO Box 1198
Fulton, KY 42041-1198
(279) 472-1638
Fax: (270) 472-6804

GRAVES
Hall Hotel, Suite 300
103 North Seventh Street
Mayfield, KY 42066
(270) 247-2862
Fax: (270) 247-2007

HICKMAN
343 Moss Avenue
PO Box 180
Clinton, KY 42031-0180
(270) 653-4338
Fax: (270) 653-2179

MCCRACKEN
Hipp Bldg., Suite 1
2855 Jackson Street
PO Box 8349
Paducah, KY 42002-8349
(270) 575-7050
Fax: (270) 575-7049

MARSHALL
211 East 7th Street
PO Box 491
Benton, KY 42025-0491
(270) 527-1395
Fax: (270) 527-2777

LOUISIANA PARISH OFFICES

ACADIA PARISH BHSF
614 North Avenue G
Mail to: PO Drawer 690
Crowley, LA 70526-0690
(318) 788-7610

ALLEN PARISH BHSF
109 North Eighth Street
PO Drawer 280
Oberlin, LA 70655-0280
(318) 335-1740

ASCENSION PARISH BHSF
515-B Marchand Drive
Mail to: PO Box 779
Donaldsonville, LA 70346-0779
(225) 474-2070
(888) 474-2070

ASSUMPTION PARISH BHSF
Lafourche Parish Medicaid
1000-E Plantation Road
Thibodaux, LA 70301
Mail to: PO Box 1038
Thibodaux, LA 70302-1038
(504) 449-5021
(800) 401-0132

AVOYELLES PARISH BHSF
113 Tucker Street
Marksville, LA 71351
(318) 253-5941
BEAUREGARD PARISH BHSF
1891 Highway 190 West
Mail to: PO Drawer 848
DeRidder, LA 70634-9990
(318) 463-6091

BIENVILLE PARISH BHSF
3020 Knight Street
Suite 260-B
Shreveport, LA 71105
(318) 263-2815
(800) 256-3068

BOSSIER PARISH BHSF
3020 Knight Street
Suite 260-B
Shreveport, LA 71105
(318) 862-9875
(800) 256-3068

CADDO PARISH BHSF
3020 Knight Street
Suite 260-B
Shreveport, LA 71105
(318) 862-9875
(800) 256-3068

CALCASIEU PARISH BHSF
2300 Broad Street
Lake Charles, LA 70601
Mail to: PO Box 3250
Lake Charles, LA 70602-3250
(318) 491-2439

CALDWELL PARISH BHSF
7112 US Highway 165
or PO Box 1329
Columbia, LA 71418
(318) 649-7915
(318) 649-2673

CAMERON PARISH BHSF
2300 Broad Street
Lake Charles, LA 70601
Mail to: PO Box 3250
Lake Charles, LA 70602-3250
(318) 491-2439

CATAHOULA PARISH BHSF
1305 Fourth Street
Jonesville, LA 71343
(318) 339-4213

CLAIBORNE PARISH BHSF
3020 Knight Street
Suite 260-B
Shreveport, LA 71105
(318) 862-9875
(800) 256-3068

CONCORDIA PARISH BHSF
27797 Highway 15
PO Box 1631
Ferriday, LA 71334
(318) 757-3202

DESOTO PARISH BHSF
430 Dixie Plaza
Natchitoches, LA 71457
(318) 357-2466
(800) 873-8987

EAST BATON ROUGE PARISH BHSF
2751 Wooddale Boulevard
PO Box 96100
Baton Rouge, LA 70896-6100
(225) 922-1542

EAST CARROLL PARISH BHSF
301 First Street
Lake Providence, LA 71254
(318) 559-2039 or (318) 559-2959

EAST FELICIANA PARISH BHSF
Feliciana Parishes Medicaid Office
12486 Feliciana Drive
Mail to: PO Box 165
Clinton, LA 70722-0165
(225) 683-4757
(800) 259-9841

EVANGELINE PARISH BHSF
1008 West LaSalle Street
Ville Platte, LA 70586
(318) 363-4262

FRANKLIN PARISH BHSF
2401 Loop Road
PO Box 760
Winnsboro, LA 71295
(318) 362-3285 or (318) 435-2106

GRANT PARISH BHSF
100 8th Street
ColFax, LA 71417
(318) 627-5388

IBERIA PARISH BHSF
322 Providence Street
PO Box 14010
New Iberia, LA 70562-4010
(318) 373-0062

IBERVILLE PARISH BHSF
24710 Plaza Drive
PO Box 269
Plaquemine, LA 70765-0269
(225) 692-7014 or (800) 631-0941

JACKSON PARISH BHSF
244 Bond Street
PO Box 490
Jonesboro, LA 71251
(318) 259-4401 or (318) 259-2411

JEFFERSON, WEST BANK PARISH BHSF
Harvey State Office Building
2150 Westbank Expway, Rm. 329
Harvey, LA 70058
Mail to: PO Box 449
Gretna, LA 70054-0449
(504) 361-6973

JEFFERSON, EAST BANK PARISH BHSF
1001 Howard Avenue10th Floor
New Orleans, LA 70113
Mail to: PO Box 60840
New Orleans, LA 70160-0840
(504) 599-0656

JEFFERSON DAVIS PARISH BHSF
742 East Plaquemine Street
PO Box 879
Jennings, LA 70546-0879
(318) 824-3694

LAFAYETTE PARISH BHSF
825 Kaliste Saloom Road
Building 6, Suite 108
PO Box 80708
Lafayette, LA 70598-0708
(318) 262-5111

LAFOURCHE PARISH BHSF
1000-E Plantation Road
Thibodaux, LA 70301
Mail to: PO Box 1038
Thibodaux, LA 70302-1038
(504) 449-5021

LASALLE PARISH BHSF
Nebo Road, Highway 127 South
PO Box 1378
Jena, LA 71342-1378
(318) 992-5320

LINCOLN PARISH BHSF
1102 East Georgia, Suite B
Ruston, LA 71270
(318) 251-2259

LIVINGSTON PARISH BHSF
1279 Del Este
Denham Springs, LA 70726
(225) 665-1899

MADISON PARISH BHSF
606 East Green Street
PO Box 1560
Tallulah, LA 71284
(318) 574-4531or (318) 574-0985

MOREHOUSE PARISH BHSF
1055 East Madison
PO Box 1488
Bastrop, LA 71221
(318) 283-0825 or (318) 362-5235

NATCHITOCHES PARISH BHSF
430 Dixie Plaza
Natchitoches, LA 71457
(Shreveport Regional Sub-office)
(318) 357-2466
(800) 873-8987

ORLEANS PARISH BHSF
1001 Howard Avenue
10th Floor
New Orleans, LA 70113
Mail to: PO Box 60840
New Orleans, LA 70160-0840
(504) 599-0656

OUACHITA PARISH BHSF
1306 North 19th Street
Monroe, LA 71201
Mail to: PO Box 1432
Monroe, LA 71210-1432
(318) 362-4113

PLAQUEMINE PARISH BHSF
251 F. Edward Hebert Boulevard
Belle Chasse, LA 70037
Mail to: PO Box 449
Gretna, LA 70054-0449
(504) 393-5805
(800) 259-5805

POINTE COUPEE PARISH BHSF
120 Alamo Street
PO Box 489
New Roads, LA 70760-0489
(225) 638-6584

RAPIDES PARISH BHSF
900 Murray Street
PO Box 551
Alexandria, LA 71309-2410
(318) 487-5137

RED RIVER PARISH BHSF
430 Dixie Plaza
Natchitoches, LA 71457
(Shreveport Regional Sub-office)
(318) 357-2466
(800) 873-8987

RICHLAND PARISH BHSF
112 Morgan Street
PO Box 837
Rayville, LA 71269-0837
(318) 728-325

SABINE PARISH BHSF
430 Dixie Plaza
Natchitoches, LA 71457
(Shreveport Regional Sub-office)
(318) 357-2466
(800) 873-8987

STREET BERNARD PARISH BHSF
1001 Howard Avenue
10th Floor
New Orleans, LA 70113
Mail to: PO Box 60840
New Orleans, LA 70160-0840
(504) 599-0656

STREET CHARLES PARISH BHSF
Tri-Parish Medicaid
421 West Airline Highway, Suite H
LaPlace, LA 70068
Mail to: PO Box 1295
LaPlace, LA 70069-1295
(504) 651-4809
(800) 788-4827

STREET HELENA PARISH BHSF
1279 Del Este
Denham Springs, LA 70726
(225) 665-1899

STREET JAMES PARISH BHSF
Tri-Parish Medicaid
421 West Airline Highway, Suite H
LaPlace, LA 70068
Mail to: PO Box 1295
LaPlace, LA 70069-1295
(504) 651-4809
(800) 788-4827

STREET JOHN PARISH BHSF
Tri-Parish Medicaid
421 West Airline Highway, Suite H
LaPlace, LA 70068
Mail to: PO Box 1295
LaPlace, LA 70069-1295
(504) 651-4809
(800) 788-4827

STREET LANDRY PARISH BHSF
1283 Service Road, Highway 167 South
Opelousas, LA 70570
(318) 942-0155

STREET MARTIN PARISH BHSF
1109 South Main Street
PO Drawer 319
Street Martinville, LA 70582-1071
(318) 394-3228

STREET MARY PARISH BHSF
15213 LA Highway 182 West
PO Box 1071
Franklin, LA 70538-1071
(318) 828-2611
(800) 351-4879

STREET TAMMANY PARISH BHSF
2000 Covington Center
Covington, LA 70433
Mail to: PO Box 788
Covington, LA 70434-0788
(504) 893-6215

TANGIPAHOA PARISH BHSF
1518 Martens Drive
Hammond, LA 70401-1600
(504) 543-4216

TENSAS PARISH BHSF
205 Twelfth Street
PO Box 6186
Street Joseph, LA 71366-6186
(318) 766-9040

TERREBONNE PARISH BHSF
5593 Highway 311
Houma, LA 70360
Mail to: PO Box 830
Houma, LA 70361-0830
(504) 873-2030

UNION PARISH BHSF
117 Marion Highway
PO Box 490
Farmerville, LA 71241
(318) 368-3166

VERMILLION PARISH BHSF
1820-A Veterans Memorial Drive
PO Drawer 1035
Abbeville, LA 70510-9115
(318) 898-2854

VERNON PARISH BHSF
1603 Boone Street
PO Box 370
Leesville, LA 71496-0370
(318) 238-7022

WASHINGTON PARISH BHSF
403 Okechobee Avenue
Bogalusa, LA 70427
(225) 732-6844

WEBSTER PARISH BHSF
3020 Knight Street
Suite 260-B
Shreveport, LA 71105
(318) 862-9875
(800) 256-3068

WEST BATON ROUGE PARISH BHSF
Iberville & West Baton Rouge Parishes Medicaid
24710 Plaza Drive
PO Box 269
Plaquemine, LA 70765-0269
(225) 692-7014 or (800) 631-0941

WEST CARROLL PARISH BHSF
702 East Jefferson Street
PO Box 728
Oak Grove, LA 71263
(318) 428-3252

WEST FELICIANA PARISH BHSF
Feliciana Parishes Medicaid Office
12486 Feliciana Drive
Clinton, LA 70722
Mail to: PO Box 165
Clinton, LA 70722-0165
(225) 683-4757
(800) 259-9841

WINN PARISH BHSF
1408 East Lafayette Street
PO Box 231
Winnfield, LA 71483
(318) 628-2746

MAINE

DHS REGIONAL OFFICES

Region I:
PORTLAND (MAIN OFFICE)
509 Forest Avenue
Portland, ME 04101
774-4581
(800) 482-7520 (Toll Free)
TTY (800) 492-0670 (Toll Free)

BIDDEFORD
208 Graham Street
Biddeford, ME 04005
282-6191
(800) 322-1919 (Toll Free)
TTY 284-9397

SANFORD
39 Wentworth Street
Sanford, ME 04073
324-9472
(800) 482-0790 (Toll Free)
TTY 324-8930

Region II:
LEWISTON (MAIN OFFICE)
200 Main Street
Lewiston, ME 04240
795-4300
(800) 482-7517 (Toll Free)
TTY 784-4421

FARMINGTON
25 Main Street
Farmington, ME 04938
778-6054
(800) 442-6382 (Toll Free)

Region III:
AUGUSTA (MAIN OFFICE)
2 Anthony Avenue
Augusta, ME 04333
624-8000
(800) 452-1926 (Toll Free)
TTY (800) 633-0770 (Toll Free)

BELFAST
55 North port Avenue
Belfast, ME 04915
338-2060

ROCKLAND
360 Old County Road
Rockland, ME 04841
596-4200
(800) 432-7802 (Toll Free)
TTY (800) 432-1680 (Toll Free)

SKOWHEGAN
140 North Avenue
Skowhegan, ME 04976
474-4800
(800) 452-4602 (Toll Free)

Region IV:
BANGOR (MAIN OFFICE)
396 Griffin Road
Bangor, ME 04401
561-4100
(800) 432-7825 (Toll Free)
TTY 945-6711

CALAIS
88 A South Street
Calais, ME 04619
454-2131
(800) 622-1400 (Toll Free)

DOVER-FOXCROFT
125 Summer Street
Dover-Foxcroft, ME 04426
564-3444
(800) 432-1641 (Toll Free)

ELLSWORTH
Short Street
Ellsworth, ME 04605
667-5361
(800) 432-7823 (Toll Free)

MACHIAS
100 Court Street
Machias, ME 04654
255-8641
(800) 432-7846 (Toll Free)

Region V:
HOULTON (MAIN OFFICE)
11 High Street
Houlton, ME 04730
532-5000
(800) 432-7338 (Toll Free)

CARIBOU
RT. 1 & 89 Access Highway
Caribou, ME 04736
Mail to: RR2, Box 8700
Caribou, ME 04736
493-4000
(800) 432-7366 (Toll Free)
TTY 493-3041

FORT KENT
92 Market Street
Fort Kent, ME 04743-1447
834-7700
(800) 432-7340 (Toll Free)

MARYLAND DEPARTMENT OF SOCIAL SERVICES

CATONSVILLE DISTRICT BRANCH OFFICE
910 Frederick Road
Catonsville, MD 21228
(410) 853-3450
Fax: (410) 853-3456
Zip Codes Serviced:
*21207-(See 21207 Directory)
21163-Granite, Woodstock
21228-Catonsville
*21043-Oella
21227-Halethorpe
*21229-Carroll
(*Indicates only portions of these zip codes are serviced by the districts)

DUNDALK DISTRICT BRANCH OFFICE
7701 Dunmanway
Dundalk, MD 21222
(410) 853-3440
Fax: (410) 853-3401
Zip Codes Serviced:
21052-Fort Howard
21219-Sparrows Point
21222-*Dundalk
(*Indicates only portions of these zip codes are serviced by the districts)

ESSEX DISTRICT BRANCH OFFICE
439 Eastern Avenue
Essex, MD 21221
(410) 853-3800
Fax: (410) 853-3850
Zip Codes Serviced:
21027-Chase
21220-Middle River
21162-White Marsh
21221-Essex
21224-*Baltimore County
(*Indicates only portions of these zip codes are serviced by the districts)

REISTERSTOWN DISTRICT BRANCH OFFICE
12035 Reisterstown Road
Reisterstown, MD 21236
(410) 853-3010
Fax: (410) 853-3069
Zip Codes Serviced:
21020-Boring
21023-Butler
21055-Garrison
21071-Glyndon
21074-*Hampstead
21117-Owings Mills
21244-(See 21207 directory)
21133-Randallstown
21136-Reisterstown
21155-Upperco
21208-Pikesville
21215-*Baltimore County
21207-*(See 21207 directory)
21244-(See 21207 directory)
(*Indicates only portions of these zip codes are serviced by the districts)

TOWSON DISTRICT BRANCH OFFICE
1 Investment Place
Towson, MD 21204
(410) 853-3346
Fax: (410) 853-3310
Zip Codes Serviced:
21013-Baldwin
21019-Bentley Springs
21021-Bradshaw
21022-Brooklandville
21030-Cockeysville
21051-Fork
21053-Freeland
21057-Glen Arm
21082-Hydes
21087-Kingsville
21092-Long Green
21093-Lutherville
21093-Timonium
21105-Maryland Line
21111-Monkton
21120-Parkton
21128-Perry Hall
21131-Phoenix
21152-Sparks
21153-Stevenson
21156-Upper Falls
21161-White Hall
21204-Towson
21206-*Raspeburg
21209-*Mt. Washington
21210-*Roland Park

21212-*Govans
21234-*Parkville
21236-Bel Air/Joppa Road
21237-*Rosedale
21239 *Small Portion
(*Indicates only portions of these zip codes are serviced by the districts)

MASSACHUSETTS

Mass Health Enrollment Center
300 Ocean Avenue, Suite 4000
Revere, MA 02151
781-485-2500

Mass Health Enrollment Center
333 Bridge Street
Springfield, MA 01103
413-785-4100

Mass Health Enrollment Center
21 Spring Street, Suite 4
Taunton, MA 02780-0771
508-828-4600

Mass Health Enrollment Center
367 East Street
Tewksbury, MA 01876-1957
978-863-9200

MICHIGAN FAMILY INDEPENDENCE AGENCY–COUNTY OFFICES

ALCONA
PO Box 586
205 North State Street
Harrisville, MI 38740
(517) 724-6291
Fax: (517) 724-5716

ALGER
101 Court Street
(906) 387-4440
Munising, MI 49862
Fax: (906) 387-4710

ALLEGAN
2233 33rd Street
Allegan, MI 49010
(616) 673-7700
Fax: (616) 673-7795

ALPENA
711 West Chisholm
Alpena, MI 49707
(517) 354-7200
Fax: (517) 354-7242

ANTRIM
PO Box 316
205 East Cayuga Street
Bellaire, MI 49615
(231) 533-8664
Fax: (231) 533-8740

ARENAC
PO Box 130
3709 Deep River Road
Standish, MI 48658
(517) 846-4551
Fax: (517) 846-4365

BARAGA
PO Box 128
17 West Broad Street
L'Anse, MI 49946
906-524-6126
Fax: 906-524-5605

BARRY
555 West Woodlawn
Hastings, MI 49058
616-948-3200
Fax: 616-948-9069

BAY
1399 West Center Road
Essexville, MI 48732
517-895-2100
517-895-2494

BENZIE
PO Box 114
488 Court Plaza
Government Center
Beulah, MI 49617
231-882-4443
Fax: 231-882-9078

BERRIEN
PO Box 1407
401 Eighth Street
Benton Harbor, MI 49023-1407
616-934-2000
Fax: 616-934-2115

BRANCH
388 KeithWilhelm Drive
Coldwater, MI 49036
517-279-4200
Fax: 517-278-5346

CALHOUN
190 East Michigan Avenue
PO Box 490
Battle Creek, MI 49016-0490
616-966-1284
Fax: 616-966-2835

CASS
325 M-62
Cassopolis, MI 49031-1056
616-445-0200
Fax: 616-445-0299

CHARLEVOI
PO Box 37
6479 M-66
Charlevoi, MI 49720
231-547-4471
Fax: 231-547-4712

CHEBOYGA
827 South Huron Street
Cheboygan, MI 49721-2209
231-627-8500
Fax: 231-627-8546

CHIPPEWA
208 Bingham Avenue
Sault Suite
Marie, MI 49783
906-632-3377
Fax: 906-635-4173

CLARE
725 Richard Dr
Harrison, MI 48625
517-539-4260
Fax: 517-539-5302

CLINTON
201 West Railroad
Street Johns, MI 48879
517-224-5500
Fax: 517-224-8717

CRAWFORD
230 Huron
PO Box 702
Grayling, MI 49738
517-348-7691
Fax: 517-348-2838

DELTA
2940 College Avenue
Escanaba, MI 49829-9596
906-786-5394
Fax: 906-786-5350

DICKINSON
1238 Carpenter Avenue
Iron Mountain, MI 49801
(906) 774-1484
Fax: (906) 774-2775

EATON
1050 Endependence Blvd
Charlotte, MI 48813
(517) 543-0860
Fax: (517) 543-5726

MINNESOTA COUNTY HEALTH & HUMAN SERVICE AGENCIES

AITKIN
204 First Street, North West
Aitkin, MN 56431-1291
General Info/Financial Services (218) 927-2141
Social Services (218) 927-3744
Fax: (218) 927-7210

ANOKA
County Government Center
2100 Third Avenue
Anoka, MN 55303-2264
General Information (612) 422-7000
Human Services Administration (612) 422-7000
Fax: (612) 422-6987
TTY (612) 323-6166

BECKER
County Annex
712 Minnesota Avenue
PO Box 1637
Detroit Lakes, MN 56501-1637
(218) 847-5628
Fax: (218) 847-6738

BELTRAMI
616 America Avenue North West
PO Box 6008
Bemidji, MN 56619-6008
General Information/Income Maintenance (218) 759-8300
Fax: (218) 759-4150

BELTRAMI (RED LAKE BRANCH)
BIA Building
PO Box 291
Red Lake, MN 56671-0291
Red Lake Branch (218) 679-3945
Fax: (218) 679-3040

BENTON COUNTY
531 Dewey Street
PO Box 740
Foley, MN 56329-0740
(320) 968-6254
Fax: (320) 968-8906
TTY: (320) 968-8842

BIG STONE COUNTY
340 North West Second Street
PO Box 338
Ortonville, MN 56278-0338
(320) 839-2555
Fax: (320) 839-3966
TTY: (320) 839-6161

BLUE EARTH
Government Center
410 South 5th Street
PO Box 3526
Mankato, MN 56002-3526
(507) 389-8319
Fax: (507) 389-8379

BROWN
1117 Center Street
PO Box 788
New Ulm, MN 56073-0788
(507) 354-8246
Fax: (507) 359-6542
TTY: (507) 359-6505

CARLTON
1215 Avenue C
Cloquet, MN 55720-1610
(218) 879-4583
Fax: (218) 879-1925

(SOUTH) CARLTON
316 Elm Street
Moose Lake, MN 55767
(218) 485-8520
Fax: (218) 485-0477

CARVER COUNTY COMMUNITY SOCIAL SERVICES
600 East Fourth Street
Chaska, MN 55318-2191
(612) 361-1600
Fax: (612) 361-1660
TTY through MN Relay System (800) 627-3529

CASS
Social Services Building
400 Michigan Avenue West
PO Box 519
Walker, MN 56484-0519
(218) 547-1340
Fax: (218) 547-1448

CHIPPEWA
Community Service Building
719 North 7th Street, Suite 200
Montevideo, MN 56265-1397
(320) 269-6401
Fax: (320) 269-6405

CHISAGO
313 North Main Street, Room 239
Center City, MN 55012-9665
(651) 257-0324
North Branch (651) 674-4433
Fax: (651) 257-0317
TTY: (651) 257-0300

CLAY
715 North 11th Street, Suite 502
Moorhead, MN 56560-2095
(218) 299-5200
Fax: (218) 299-7515
TTY: (218) 299-5230

CLEARWATER
216 Park Avenue North
PO Box X
Bagley, MN 56621-0682
(218) 694-6164
Fax: (218) 694-3535

COOK
11 West 2nd Street
PO Box 1150
Grand Marais, MN 55604-1150
(218) 387-3000 ext 119
Fax: (218) 387-3020

COTTONWOOD
11 Fourth Street
PO Box 9
Windom, MN 56101-0009
(507) 831-1891
Fax: (507) 831-0126

CROW WING
322 Laurel Street
PO Box 686
Brainerd, MN 56401-0686
(218) 828-3966
Fax: (218) 828-2927

DAKOTA
60 East Marie Avenue, Suite 214
West Saint Paul, MN 55118-3488
(651) 450-2611
Fax: (651) 450-2709

DODGE
PO Box 278
Mantorville, MN 55955-0278
(507) 635-6170
Fax: (507) 635-6186
TTY: (507) 635-6200

DOUGLAS
809 Elm Street
PO Box 3001
Alexandria, MN 56308
(320) 762-2302
Fax: (320) 762-3833

FARIBAULT & MARTIN
Human Services of Faribault & Martin Counties
115 West First Street
Fairmont, MN 56031-1815
(507) 238-4757
Fax: (507) 238-1574
Community Social Services (507) 526-3265

FILLMORE
PO Box 550
Preston, MN 55965-0550
(507) 765-2175
Fax: (507) 765-3895

FREEBORN
203 West Clark Street
PO Box 1246
Albert Lea, MN 56007-1246
(507) 337-5400
Fax: (507) 337-5498
TTY: (507) 337-5519

GOODHUE
426 West Avenue
PO Box 31
Red Wing, MN 55066-0031
(651) 385-3232
Fax: (651) 385-3191
Fax: (651) 385-3205
TTY: (651) 385-3190

GRANT
28 Central South
PO Box 1006
Elbow Lake, MN 56531-1006
(218) 685-4417
Fax: (218) 685-4978

HENNEPIN
A-2303 Government Center
300 South 6th Street
Minneapolis, MN 55487-0233
(612) 348-3000
Fax: (612) 348-8228

HOUSTON
304 South Marshall
PO Box 310
Caledonia, MN 55921-0310
(507) 724-5811
Fax: (507) 724-3990

HUBBARD
301 Court Street
Park Rapids, MN 56470-1483
(218) 732-1451
Fax: (218) 732-3231

ISANTI
553 18th Avenue South West
Cambridge, MN 55008-9386
(612) 689-1711
Fax: (612) 689-9877

ITASCA
1209 South East 2nd Avenue
Grand Rapids, MN 55744-3983
(218) 327-2941
Social Services (218) 327-2981
Fax: (218) 327-5547
IMCare Fax: (218) 326-7708
TTY: (218) 327-5549

JACKSON
310 Sherman Street
PO Box 67
Jackson, MN 56143-0067
(507) 847-4000

KANABEC
PO Box 180
Mora, MN 55051-1316
(320) 679-6350
Fax: (320) 679-6351

KANDIYOHI
1900 Highway 294 NE, Suite 1020
Willmar, MN 56201-9423
(320) 231-6232
Fax: (320) 231-6285

KITTSON
410 South 5th Street
PO Box 160
Hallock, MN 56728-0160
(218) 843-2689
Fax: (218) 843-2607

KOOCHICHING
1000-5th Street
International Falls, MN 56649-2485
(218) 283-8405
Fax: (218) 283-6213

KOOCHICHING NORTH HOME BRANCH (SATELLITE OFFICE)
County Office Building
Northome, MN 56661
(218) 897-5275

LAC QUI PARLE
930 First Avenue
PO Box 7
Madison, MN 56256-0007
(320) 598-7594
Fax: (320) 598-7597

LAKE
616 Third Avenue
Two Harbors, MN 55616-1560
(218) 834-8400
Fax: (218) 834-8412

LAKE OF THE WOODS
905 South East First Street
PO Box G-200
Baudette, MN 56623-0200
(218) 634-2642
Fax: (218) 634-4520

LESUEUR
88 South Park Avenue
LeCenter, MN 56057-1646
(507) 357-2251
Fax: (507) 357-6122

LINCOLN
319 North Rebecca Street
PO Box 44
Ivanhoe, MN 56142-0044
General Information, Voice/TTY (507) 694-1452
Fax: (507) 694-1859

LYON
607 West Main Street
Marshall, MN 56258-3099
(507) 537-6747
Fax: (507) 537-6088
TTY: (507) 532-1250

MCLEOD
Health & Human Services Building
1805 Ford Avenue North
Glencoe, MN 55336-0130
General Information-Voice/TTY (320) 864-3144
Fax: (320) 864-5265

MAHNOMEN
311 North Main Street
PO Box 460
Mahnomen, MN 56557-0460
(218) 935-2568
Fax: (218) 935-5459

MARSHALL
208 East Colvin Avenue
Warren, MN 56762-1695
(218) 745-5124
Fax: (218) 745-5260

FARIBAULT & MARTIN
115 West First Street
Fairmont, MN 56031-1815
(507) 238-4757
Fax: (507) 238-1574
Community Social Services (507) 526-3265

MEEKER
114 North Holcombe Avenue, Suite 180
Litchfield, MN 55355-2273
(320) 693-5300
Fax: (320) 693-5344

MILLE LACS
635 2nd Street South East
Milaca, MN 56353-1396
(320) 983-8208
Fax: (320) 983-8306

MORRISON
Government Center
213 SouthEast First Avenue
Little Falls, MN 56345-3196
(651) 632-2951
Fax: (651) 632-0225

MOWER
1005 North Main Street
Austin, MN 55912-3317
(507) 437-9700
Fax: (507) 437-9721

MURRAY
3095 20th Street
Slayton, MN 56172-1493
(507) 836-6144
Fax: (507) 836-8841

NICOLLET
108 South Minnesota Avenue, Suite 200
Saint Peter, MN 56082-2516
(507) 931-6800
Fax: (507) 931-9562

NICOLLET (NORTH MANKATO BRANCH OFFICE)
2070 Howard Drive
Mankato, MN 56003-1527
(507) 387-4556
Fax: (507) 387-2918

NOBLES
901 Fourth Avenue
PO Box 189
Worthington, MN 56187-0189
(507) 372-2157
Fax: (507) 372-5094

NORMAN
County Office Building
15-2nd Avenue East, Room 108
Ada, MN 56510-1389
(218) 784-7136
Fax: (218) 784-7142

OLMSTED
51 4th Street South East
Rochester, MN 55904-3711
(507) 285-8382
Social Services (507) 285-7009
Fax: (507) 287-2434

OTTER TAIL
505 South Court Street
Fergus Falls, MN 56537-2703
(218) 739-4491
Fax: (218) 739-2909

PENNINGTON
318 North Knight Avenue
PO Box 340
Thief River Falls, MN 56701-0340
(218) 681-2880
Fax: (218) 683-7013

PINE
15 6th Street
PO Box 110
Pine City, MN 55063-0110
(320) 629-6781
(800) 450-7463
Fax: (320) 629-7319
TTY: (800) 627-3529

SANDSTONE BRANCH
PO Box 100
Sandstone, MN 55072-0100
(320) 245-2268
(800) 450-7263
Fax: (320) 245-2268

PIPESTONE
121 West Main
PO Box 157
Pipestone, MN 56164-0157
(507) 825-6720
Fax: (507) 825-6727

POLK FOSSTON BRANCH
108 2nd Street North West
Fosston, MN 56542-1229
(218) 435-1585
Fax: (218) 435-1552

POLK COUNTY SOCIAL SERVICE CENTER
612 North Broadway, Suite 110
Crookston, MN 56716-1452
(218) 281-3127
Fax: (218) 281-3926
TTY: (218) 281-3127 ext 103

CROOKSTON BRANCH
Income Maintenance Unit
223 East 7th Street Suite 109
Crookston, MN 56716-1498
Income Maintenance (218) 281-7329
Fax: (218) 281-7347

EAST GRAND FORKS BRANCH
1622 Central Avenue NE
East Grand Forks, MN 56721-1335
(218) 773-2431
Fax: (218) 773-3602

POPE
130 Minnesota Avenue East
Glenwood, MN 56334-1628
General Information (218) 634-5750
Fax: (218) 634-0164

RAMSEY
160 East Kellogg Boulevard
Street Paul, MN 55101-1494
General Information (651) 266-4444
Fax: (651) 266-4439

RED LAKE
125 Edward Avenue
PO Box 356
Red Lake Falls, MN 56750-0356
General Information (218) 253-4131
Fax: (218) 253-2926

REDWOOD
302 East Third Street
PO Box 510
Redwood Falls, MN 56283
General Information (507) 637-4050

RENVILLE
301 South Seventh Street
Olivia, MN 56277-1301
General Information (320) 523-2202
Fax: (320) 523-3565

RICE
320 NW Third Street #B
PO Box 718
Faribault, MN 55021-0718
General Information (507) 332-6115
Fax: (507) 332-6247
TTY: (507) 332-6248

ROCK
2 Roundwind Road
PO Box 715
Luverne, MN 56156-0715
General Information (507) 283-5070
Fax: (507) 283-5074
TTY: (507) 283-5070

ROSEAU
300-6th Street South West
Roseau, MN 56751-1451
General Information (218) 463-2411
Fax: (218) 463-3872

SAINT LOUIS
Government Services Center
320 West 2nd Street
Duluth, MN 55802-1495
General Info (218) 726-2000
Fax: (218) 726-2253
TTY: (218) 726-2222

SAINT LOUIS (VIRGINIA OFFICE)
Northland Office Center, PO Box 1148
Virginia, MN 55792-1148
(218) 749-7100
(218) 749-7123

SAINT LOUIS (ELY OFFICE)
118 South Fourth Avenue, East
Ely, MN 55731-1402
(218) 365-6151
Fax: (218) 365-6453

SAINT LOUIS (HIBBING OFFICE)
2534 East Beltline
Hibbing, MN 55746-2302
(218) 262-6000
Fax: (218) 262-6049

SCOTT
Courthouse, Room 300
428 Holmes Street South
Shakopee, MN 55379-1375
General Information (612) 445-7751
Fax: (612) 496-8430
Fax: (612) 496-8551

SHERBURNE
Becker Branch Office
13122 1st Street
Becker, MN 55308-9320
For people in Becker (800) 821-9719
For people in Becker (612) 441-1880
Unspecified (612) 261-5048
Fax: (612) 261-4550

SHERBURNE
13880 Highway 10
Elk River, MN 55330-4600
(800) 433-5239 or (612) 241-2600
Fax: (612) 241-2698

SIBLEY
112 Fifth Street
Gaylord, MN 55334-0237
General Information-Voice/TTY (507) 237-4000
Fax: (507) 237-4031

STEARNS
Administration Center
705 Courthouse Square
PO Box 1107
Street Cloud, MN 56302-1107
(800) 450-3663
(320) 656-6000
Fax: (320) 656-6253
TTY: (320) 656-6204

STEARNS (BELGRADE OFFICE)
615 Washburn Avenue South
PO Box 39
Belgrade, MN 56312
(320) 254-3694
Fax: (320) 254-3770

STEARNS (MELROSE OFFICE)
114 South 1st Avenue West
PO Box 128
Melrose, MN 56352
(320) 256-3308
Fax: (320) 256-7666

STEELE
630 Florence Avenue
PO Box 890
Owatonna, MN 55060-0890
General Information 507-444-7500
Fax: 507-451-5947

STEVENS
400 Colorado Avenue
PO Box 530-HS
Morris, MN 56267-0530
(320) 589-7400
Fax: (320) 589-3972

SWIFT
109-12th Street South
PO Box 208
Benson, MN 56215-0208
(320) 843-3160
Fax: (320) 843-4582

TODD
Courthouse Annex
212 2nd Avenue South
Long Prairie, MN 56347-1640
(320) 732-4500
(888) 838-4066
Fax: (320) 732-4540

TRAVERSE
203 8th Street North
PO Box 46
Wheaton, MN 56296
(320) 563-8255
Fax: (320) 563-4230

WABASHA
625 Jefferson Avenue
Wabasha, MN 55981-1589
(651) 565-3351
Fax: (651) 565-3084

WADENA
124 1st Street South East
Wadena, MN 56482-1553
(218) 631-7605
Fax: (218) 631-7616

WASECA
123-3rd Avenue North West
Waseca, MN 56093-2498
(507-835-0560
Fax: (507) 835-0566

WASHINGTON
14900-61st Street North
PO Box 30
Stillwater, MN 55082-0030
(651) 430-6455
Fax: (651) 430-6605

WATONWAN
720-1st Avenue South
PO Box 31
Street James, MN 56081-0031
(507) 375-3294
Fax: (507) 375-7359

WILKIN
300 5th Street South
PO Box 369
Breckenridge, MN 56520-0369
(218) 643-8561
Fax: (218) 643-2230

WINONA
County Office Building
202 W 3rd St
Winona, MN 55987-3146
(507) 457-6200
Fax: (507) 454-9382

WRIGHT
10 2nd Street NW, Room 300
Buffalo, MN 55313-1191
(612) 682-7414
Social Services & Community Health (612) 682-7400
Fax: (612) 682-7701

YELLOW MEDICINE
415-9th Avenue
Granite Falls, MN 56241-1367
(320) 564-2211
Fax: (320) 564-4165

MISSISSIPPI

REGION I-EAST
Counties:
Chickasaw, Clay, Itawamba, Lee, Monroe, Pontotoc, Prentiss, Tishomingo, Union, Webster

PRENTISS COUNTY DHS
PO Box 728
Booneville, MS 38829
662-728-8020
Fax: 662-728-0940

REGION I-WEST
Counties:
Alcorn, Benton, Calhoun, Desoto, Lafayette, Marshall, Panola, Tate, Tippah, Tunica

LAFAYETTE COUNTY DHS
PO Box 1027
Oxford, MS 38655
662-234-1863
Fax: 662-236-0230

REGION II
Counties:
East Bolivar, West Bolivar, Coahoma, Grenada, Humphreys, Quitman, Sunflower, Tallahatchie, Washington, Yalobusha

GRENADA COUNTY DHS
1241 South Mound Street
Grenada, MS 38902
662-226-1351
Fax: 662-226-1432

REGION III
Counties:
Attala, Carroll, Holmes, Issaquena, Leake, Leflre, Madison, Montgomery, Rankin, Scott, Sharkey, Yazoo

SHARKEY COUNTY DHS
PO Box 488
Rolling Fork, MS 39159
662-873-6144
Fax: 662-873-6145

REGION IV
Counties:
Choctaw, Clarke, Jasper, Kemper, Lauderdale, Lowndes, Neshoba, Newton, Noxubee, Oktibbeha, Smith, Wayne, Winston

LAUDERDALE COUNTY DHS
PO Box 910
Meridian, MS 39302
601-486-2992
Fax: 601-486-2996

MISSOURI HOME AND COMMUNITY SERVICES REGIONS

HOME AND COMMUNITY SERVICES REGIONS
PO Box 1337
615 Howerton Court
Jefferson City, MO 65102
Phone: (573) 751-3082
Fax: (573) 751-8687

REGIONAL OFFICES
REGION 1
149 Park Central Square
Springfield, MO 65806
(417) 895-6456
Fax: (417) 895-1341

REGION 2
130 South Frederick
Cape Girardeau, MO 63701
(573) 290-5781
Fax: (573) 290-5650

Region 3-7
Suite 405, State Office
615 East 13th Street
Kansas City, MO 64106
(816) 889-3100
Fax: (816) 889-2004

Region 4
525 Jules Street, Room 319
Street Joseph, MO 64501
(660) 387-2100
Fax: (660) 387-2110

REGION 5-6
1500 Vandiver Drive Suite 102
Columbia, MO 65202
(573) 882-9474
Fax: (573) 884-4884

REGION 8-9
Wainwright Building
111 North 7th Street, 4th Floor
Street Louis, MO 63101
(314) 340-7300
Fax: (314) 340-3415

MISSOURI INSTITUTIONAL SERVICES REGIONS

Institutional Services
PO Box 1337
615 Howerton Court
Jefferson City, MO 65102
Phone: (573) 751-3082
Fax: (573) 751-8687

Regional Offices

REGION 1
149 Park Central Square
Springfield, MO 65806
(417) 895-6435
Fax: (417) 895-6444

REGION 2
1903 North wood Drive
PO Box 1207
Poplar Bluff, MO 63901
(573) 840-9580
Fax: (573) 840-9586

REGION 3
4th Floor, State Office Building
615 East 13th Street
Kansas City, MO 64106
(816) 889-2818
Fax: (816) 889-2161

REGION 4
1115 West Grand
PO Box 633
Cameron, MO 64429
(816) 632-6541
Fax: (816) 632-1810

REGION 5
311 North Rollins
Macon, MO 63552
(660) 385-5763
Fax: (660) 385-4706

REGION 6
3418 Knipp Drive
POBox 915
Jefferson City, MO 65102
(573) 751-2270
Fax: (573) 526-1269

REGION 7
Wainwright Building, Room 500
111 North 7th Street
Street Louis, MO 63101
(314) 340-7360
Fax: (314) 340-3414

MONTANA HUMAN AND COMMUNITY SERVICES DIVISION

BEAVERHEAD
2 South Pacific #9
Dillon, MT 59725
(406) 683-2142
Fax: (406) 683-5080

BIG HORN
23 West 8th
PO Box 426
Hardin, MT 59034
(406) 665-1906
Fax: (406) 665-3675

BLAINE
Courthouse Annex
PO Box 1088
Chinook, MT 59523
(406) 357-2276
Fax: (406) 357-2436

BROADWATER
124 North Cedar
Townsend, MT 59644
(406) 222-8000
Fax: (406) 222-5742

CARBON
206 North Broadway
PO Box 670
Red Lodge, MT 59068
406-446-1302
Fax: 406-446-9155

CASCADE
1601 2nd Avenue North 3rd Floor
PO Box 1546
Great Falls, MT 59401
(406) 454-5640
Fax: (406) 454-5697

CHOUTEAU
1020 13th Street
PO Box 459
Fort Benton, MT 59442
(406) 622-5432
Fax: (406) 622-3848

CUSTER
Courthouse Basement
1010 Main Street
Miles City, MT 59301
(406) 233-3334
Fax: (406) 233-3449
Counties: Custer, Powder River, Garfield, McCone, Prairie

DAWSON
121 South Douglas
Glendive, MT 59330
(406) 377-4314
Fax: (406) 377-5917

DEER LODGE
307 East Park, Rm 305
Anaconda, MT 59711
(406) 563-3448 (Deer Lodge and Powell)
(406) 859-0009 (Granite)
Fax: (406) 563-7279 (Deer Lodge)
Fax: (406) 846-3257 (Powell)
Fax: (406) 859-3817 (Granite)
Counties: Deer Lodge, Powell, Granite

FALLON
10 West Fallon Avenue
PO Box 759
Baker, MT 59313
(406) 778-2883
Fax: (406) 778-2815
Counties: Fallon, Carter, Wibaux

FERGUS
300 1st Avenue North Suite 201
Lewistown, MT 59457
(406) 538-7468
Fax: (406) 538-8419
Counties: Fergus, Musselshell, Judith Basin, Petroleum, Wheatland,
        Golden Valley

FLATHEAD
2282 Highway 93 South
PO Box 1096
Kalispell, MT 59903
(406) 751-5900 main number
(406) 751-5921 direct number
Fax: (406) 751-5929

GALLATIN
237 West Main
Bozeman, MT 59715
(406) 582-3010
Fax: (406) 582-3114

GLACIER
101 East Main
PO Box 3025
Browning, MT 59417
(406) 338-5131
Fax: (406) 338-7769

HILL
Courthouse
302 4th Avenue
Havre, MT 59501
(406) 265-4348
Fax: (406) 265-6919

JEFFERSON
PO Box 836
114 South Washington
Boulder, MT 59632
(406) 225-4045
Fax: (406) 225-4145

LAKE
826 Shoreline Drive
Polson, MT 59860
(406) 883-7820
Fax: (406) 883-5320

LEWIS & CLARK
PO Box 202959
3075 North Montana Avenue
Helena, MT 59620-2959
(406) 444-1700
Fax: (406) 444-1751

LINCOLN
117 Commerce Way
Libby, MT 59923
(406) 293-3791
Fax: (406) 293-5549

MADISON
313 East Idaho
PO Box 75
Virginia City, MT 59923
(406) 843-5324
Fax: (406) 843-5325

MISSOULA
301 West Alder
Missoula, MT 59802
(406) 523-4994 voice mail
(406) 523-4950 phone
Fax: (406) 721-4527 (Missoula)
Fax: (406) 822-3217 (Mineral)
Counties: Missoula, Mineral

PARK
220 East Park
Livingston, MT 59047
(406) 222-8000
Fax: (406) 222-5742 (Park)
Fax: (406) 547-3388 (Meagher)
Counties: Park, Meagher

PONDERA
Courthouse
20 4th Avenue SW
Conrad, MT 59425
(406) 278-4020 (Pondera)
(406) 466-5721 (Teton)
(406) 434-2371 (Toole)
Fax: (406) 278-4074 (Pondera)
Fax: (406) 466-2349 (Teton)
Fax: (406) 434-7293 (Toole)
Counties: Pondera, Teton, Toole

RAVALLI
310 North 3rd Street
Hamilton, MT 59840
(406) 363-1944
Fax: (406) 363-2138

RICHLAND
221 5th Street South West
Sidney, MT 59270
(406) 482-2282
Fax: (406) 482-2015

ROOSEVELT (WOLF POINT OFFICE)
Courthouse Building
Wolf Point, MT 59201
(406) 653-1210 (Roosevelt, Sheridan, Daniels)
Fax: (406) 653-2057 (Roosevelt, Sheridan, Daniels)

ROOSEVELT (SHERIDAN, DANIELS OFFICE)
100 West Laurel Avenue
PO Box 413
Plentywood, MT 59254
(406) 653-1210 (Roosevelt, Sheridan, Daniels)
Fax: (406) 653-2057 (Roosevelt, Sheridan, Daniels)

ROSEBUD
1093 Main Street
PO Box 5016
Forsyth, MT 59327
(406) 356-2563
Fax: (406) 356-7166
Counties: Rosebud, Treasure

SANDERS
Courthouse 111 Main St
PO Box 519
Thompson Falls, MT 59873
(406) 827-4395
Fax: (406) 827-4388 and (406) 827-9870

SILVER BOW
700 Casey Street
Butte, MT 59701
(406) 496-4900
Fax: (406) 496-4901

STILLWATER
PO Box 928
43 North 4th Street
Columbus, MT 59019
(406) 322-5331
Fax: (406) 322-4076
Counties: Stillwater, Sweet Grass

VALLEY
PO Box 9
Courthouse Annex
501 Court Square
Glasgow, MT 59230
(406) 228-8221 ext 50
Fax: (406) 228-4030 (Valley)
Fax: (406) 654-2254 (Phillips)
Counties: Valley, Phillips

YELLOWSTONE
111 North 31st Street
Billings, MT 59101
(406) 256-0274
Fax: (406) 256-6996

NEBRASKA DEPARTMENT OF HEALTH AND HUMAN SERVICES

ADAMS COUNTY-HASTINGS
Courthouse Annex
5th and Denver Streets
PO Box 2005
Hastings, NE 68901-2005
Phone: (402) 462-1800 or (800) 557-8544

REGIONAL CENTER
4200 West 2nd Street
PO Box 579
Hastings, NE 68901-0579
Phone: (402) 462-1971

ANTELOPE COUNTY-NELIGH
Courthouse
501 Main Street
PO Box 104
Neligh, NE 68756-0104
Phone: (402) 887-4196 or (402) 887-4197

ARTHUR COUNTY-ARTHUR
See Keith County

BANNER COUNTY-HARRISBURG
See Scotts Bluff County

BLAINE COUNTY-BREWSTER
See Custer County

BOONE COUNTY-ALBION
Courthouse
222 South 4th Street, Room 10
Albion, NE 68620
Phone: (402) 395-5036

BOX BUTTE COUNTY-ALLIANCE
PO Box 759
624 Yellowstone
Alliance, NE 69301
Phone: (308) 763-2900, (800) 843-1407

BOYD COUNTY-BUTTE
See Holt County

BROWN COUNTY-AINSWORTH
Courthouse
148 West 4th Street
Ainsworth, NE 69210
Phone: (402) 387-2523

BUFFALO COUNTY-KEARNEY
24 West 16th Street
PO Box 218
Kearney, NE 68848
Phone: (308) 865-5592, (800) 779-4855

BURT COUNTY-TEKAMEH
Courthouse
111 North 13th Street
Tekamah, NE 68061
Phone: (402) 374-2332

BUTLER COUNTY-DAVID CITY
284 North 9th Street
David City, NE 68632-2020
Phone: (402) 367-6021, (402) 367-6022, or (800) 576-5212

CASS COUNTY-PLATTSMOUTH
546 Avenue A
Plattsmouth, NE 68048
Phone: (402) 296-0000, (800) 776-1188

CEDAR COUNTY-HARTINGTON
Courthouse
Hartington, NE 68739
Phone: (402) 254-7426

CHASE COUNTY-IMPERIAL
Nebraska Department of Health and Human Services
130 West 4th
PO Box 1269
Imperial, NE 69033
Phone: (308) 882-4791, (308) 882-4816

CHERRY COUNTY-VALENTINE
Nebraska Department of Health and Human Services
Courthouse
365 North Main Street, Suite 5
Valentine, NE 69201
Phone: (402) 376-1790

CHEYENNE COUNTY-SIDNEY
Courthouse
10th and King
PO Box 357
Sidney, NE 69162
Phone: (308) 254-6900, (800) 643-7415

CLAY COUNTY-CLAY CENTER
Courthouse
111 West Fairfield
PO Box 203
Clay Center, NE 68933
Phone: (402) 762-3465, (402) 762-3318
Also serves Nuckolls County

COLF COUNTY-SCHUYLER
See Platte County

CUMING COUNTY-WEST POINT
Courthouse, Room 53
200 South Lincoln
West Point, NE 68788
Phone: (402) 372-6014

CUSTER COUNTY-BROKEN BOW
1030 South "D" Street
PO Box 508
Broken Bow, NE 68822
Phone: (308) 872-6700, (800) 497-1515

DAKOTA COUNTY-DAKOTA CITY
1601 Broadway
PO Box 474
Dakota City, NE 68731
Phone: (402) 987-3445

DAWES COUNTY-CHADRON
1201 West 8th Street
PO Box 310
Chadron, NE 69337
Phone: (308) 432-6151, (800) 559-9718

DAWSON COUNTY-LEXINGTON
Courthouse
7th and Washington, Box E
Lexington, NE 68850
Phone: (308) 324-6633, (800) 778-1613

DEUEL COUNTY-CHAPPELL
See Cheyenne County

DIXON COUNTY-PONCA
See Dakota County

DODGE COUNTY-FREMONT
124 East 5th Street
PO Box 770
Fremont, NE 68026-0770
Phone: (402) 727-3200, (800) 467-9922

DOUGLAS COUNTY-OMAHA
1313 Farnam-on-the-Mall, 3rd Floor
Omaha, NE 68102-1870
Phone: (402) 595-2850

DUNDY COUNTY-BENKELMAN
123 West 6th
Benkelman, NE 69021
Direct calls and mail to Chase County

FILLMORE COUNTY-GENEVA
900 "G" Street
PO Box 308
Geneva, NE 68361
Phone: (402) 759-3718

FRANKLIN COUNTY-FRANKLIN
Courthouse
405 15th Avenue
Franklin, NE 68939
Direct calls and mail to Buffalo County office

FRONTIER COUNTY-STOCKVILLE
Frontier County Courthouse
Stockville, NE 69042
Direct calls and mail to Red Willow County

FURNAS COUNTY-BEAVENUER CITY
Courthouse
Beaver City, NE 68926
Direct calls and mail to Red Willow County

GAGE COUNTY-BEATRICE
Route 2, Box 401
Beatrice, NE 68310
Phone: (402) 223-6000, (800) 554-9123

GARDEN COUNTY-OSHKOSH
Courthouse
Oshkosh, NE 69154
Direct calls and mail to Morrill County

GARFIELD COUNTY-BURWELL
See Valley County

GOSPER COUNTY-ELWOOD
See Dawson County

GRANT COUNTY-HYANNIS
Courthouse
Hyannis, NE 69350
Direct calls and mail to Hooker County

GREELEY COUNTY-GREELEY
See Valley County

HALL COUNTY-GRAND ISLAND
116 South Pine Street
PO Box 2440
Grand Island, NE 68802-2440
Phone: (308) 385-6100

HAMILTON COUNTY-AURORA
See Hall County

HARLAN COUNTY-ALMA
See Phelps County

HAYES COUNTY-HAYES CENTER
See Chase County
Hitchcock County-Trenton
See Red Willow County

HOLT COUNTY-O'NEILL
Courthouse Annex
128 North 6th Street
PO Box 669
O'Neill, NE 68763
Phone: (402) 336-2750

HOWARD COUNTY-STREET PAUL
See Hall County

JEFFERSON COUNTY–FAIRBURY
PO Box 556
Fairbury, NE 68352
(402) 729-6168

JOHNSON COUNTY-TECUMSEH
Courthouse
PO Box 839
Tecumseh, NE 68450
Phone: (402) 335-4102
Also serves Pawnee County

KEARNEY COUNTY-MINDEN
See Buffalo County

KEITH COUNTY-OGALLALA
201 East 5th
Ogallala, NE 69153
Phone: (308) 284-8080 or (308) 284-8081 or (800) 778-1614
Fax: (308) 284-8083

KEYA PAHA COUNTY-SPRINGVIEW
See Rock County

KIMBALL COUNTY-KIMBALL
Courthouse
114 East 3rd
Kimball, NE 69145
Direct calls and mail to Cheyenne County

KNOX COUNTY-CENTER
Courthouse
Center, NE 68724
Phone: (402) 288-4291

LANCASTER COUNTY-LINCOLN
1050 "N" Street
Lincoln, NE 68508
Phone: (402) 471-7000

LINCOLN REGIONAL CENTER
PO Box 94949
Lincoln, NE 68509-4949
Phone: (402) 471-4444

LINCOLN COUNTY-NORTH PLATTE
Craft State Office Building
200 South Silber
North Platte, NE 69101
Phone: (308) 535-8200, (800) 778-1611

LOGAN COUNTY-STAPLETON
See Lincoln County

LOUP COUNTY-TAYLOR
See Valley County

MCPHERSON COUNTY-TRYON
See Lincoln County

MADISON COUNTY-MADISON
Nebraska Department of Health and Human Services
209 North 5th Street
PO Box 339
Norfolk, NE 68702
Phone: (402) 370-3132, (800) 782-8844

NORFOLK REGIONAL CENTER
PO Box 1209
Norfolk, NE 68702-1209
Phone: (402) 370-3400

MERRICK COUNTY-CENTRAL CITY
See Hall County

MORRILL COUNTY-BRIDGEPORT
208 East 6th Street
PO Box 669
Bridgeport, NE 69336
Phone: (308) 262-1900, (800) 316-0039

NANCE COUNTY–FULLERTON
209 Esther Street
Fullerton, NE 68638
Direct mail to Boone County
Phone: (308) 536-2511

NELSON
Courthouse
Nelson, NE 68961
Direct calls and mail to Clay County

NEBRASKA CITY
1102 3rd Avenue
Nebraska City, NE 68410
Phone: (402) 873-6671, (800) 884-6411

PAWNEE COUNTY-PAWNEE CITY
See Johnson County

PERKINS COUNTY-GRANT
See Keith County

PHELPS COUNTY–HOLDREGE
Courthouse
701 Fifth Avenue
PO Box 168
Holdrege, NE 68949
Phone: (308) 995-8658

PIERCE COUNTY-PIERCE
Courthouse
111 West Court, #15
Pierce, NE 68767-1224
Phone: (402) 329-4927

PLATTE COUNTY-COLUMBUS
2365 39th Avenue-
Columbus, NE 68601
Phone: (402) 564-1113, (800) 330-0755

POLK COUNTY-OSCEOLA
See York County for residents with mailing addresses in Polk, Stromsburg, Benedict, Silver Creek, Clarks, and Gresham
Direct mail to York County

RED WILLOW COUNTY-MCCOOK
1700 North Highway 83
PO Box 1177
McCook, NE 69001
Phone: (308) 345-8420, (800) 778-1612

RICHARDSON COUNTY-FALLS CITY
Courthouse
1700 Stone Street
Falls City, NE 68355
Phone: (402) 245-4431

ROCK COUNTY-BASSETT
See Brown County

SALINE COUNTY-WILBER
Courthouse
215 South Court
PO Box 576
Wilber, NE 68465
Phone: (402) 821-2081, (800) 557-8511

SARPY COUNTY-PAPILLION
1269 Golden Gate Drive
Papillion, NE 68046
Phone: (402) 595-2600

SAUNDERS COUNTY-WAHOO
355 East 4th Street
Wahoo, NE 68066
Phone: (402) 443-4252, (800) 755-1333

SCOTTS BLUFF COUNTY-GERING
1030 "N" Street
PO Box 540
Gering, NE 69341
Phone: (308) 436-6500

SEWARD COUNTY-SEWARD
320 South 14th
Seward, NE 68434
Phone: (402) 643-6614
Fax: (402) 643-6552

SHERIDAN COUNTY-RUSHVILLE
Roads Department Building
PO Box 565
Rushville, NE 69360
Phone: (308) 327-2455

SHERMAN COUNTY-LOUP CITY
See Custer County

SIOUX COUNTY-HARRISON
See Dawes County

STANTON COUNTY-STANTON
See Madison County

THAYER COUNTY-HEBRON
Courthouse
225 North 4th Street
PO Box 24
Hebron, NE 68370
Phone: (402) 768-0400

THOMAS COUNTY-THEDFORD
See Hooker County

THURSTON COUNTY-PENDER
415 Main Street
PO Box 340
Pender, NE 68047
Phone: (402) 385-2571, (402) 385-3021, (402) 385-3022

VALLEY COUNTY-ORD
213 South 15th Street
PO Box 149
Ord, NE 68862
Phone: (308) 728-3685

WASHINGTON COUNTY-BLAIR
Courthouse
1555 Colf Street
Blair, NE 68008
Phone: (402) 426-2329

WAYNE COUNTY-WAYNE
R.R. 1, Centennial Road
PO Box 285
Wayne, NE 68787
Phone: (402) 375-7050

WEBSTER COUNTY-RED CLOUD
Courthouse
225 West 6th
Red Cloud, NE 68970
Direct calls and mail to Adams County

WHEELER COUNTY-BARTLETT
See Valley County

YORK COUNTY-YORK
2329 Nebraska Avenue
York, NE 68467
Phone: (402) 362-4471, (800) 627-3411
Also serves Polk County for residents with mailing addresses in Polk,
Stromsburg, Benedict, Silver Creek, Clarks, and Gresham

NEVADA

STATE WELFARE DISTRICT OFFICES

CARSON CITY*
755 North Roop Street
Carson City, NV 89710
(775) 687-8994 Medicaid

ELKO
850 Elm Street
Elko, NV 89801
(775) 738-2531

ELY
725 Avenue K
Ely, NV 89301
(775) 286-1650

FALLON
1735 Kaiser Street
Fallon, NV 89406
(775) 423-3161

HAWTHORNE
100 "C" Street
Hawthorne, NV 89415
(775) 945-3602

HENDERSON
145 Panama Street
Henderson, NV 89015
(702) 486-6748

LAS VEGAS (BELROSE OFFICE)
700 Belrose Street
Las Vegas, NV 89158
(702) 486-5270 Medicaid

LAS VEGAS (CHARLESTON OFFICE)
3700 East Charleston Boulevard
Las Vegas, NV 89158
(702) 486-4520

LAS VEGAS OWENS OFFICE
1040 West Owens Avenue
Las Vegas, NV 89158
(702) 486-5040

LOVELOCK
535 Western Avenue
Lovelock, NV 89419
(775) 273-7157

RENO
1350 East Ninth Street
Reno, NV 89512
(775) 688-2200

RENO*
560 Mill Street, Suite 350
Reno, NV 89502
(775) 688-2811

TONOPAH
1100 Erie Main Street
Tonopah, NV 89049
(775) 482-6626

WINNEMUCCA
501 Bridge Street
Winnemucca, NV 89445
(775) 623-6557

YERINGTON
14 Pacific Street
Yerington, NV 89447
(775) 463-3151
* Indicaites Medicaid staff locations at district office sites

NEW HAMPSHIRE

BERLIN
219 Main Street
Berlin, NH 03570-0684
(603) 752-7800
(800) 972-6111

CLAREMONT
17 Water Street
Claremont, NY 03743-0870
(603) 542-9544
(800) 982-1001

CONCORD
40 Terrill Park Drive, Unit 1
Concord, NH 03301-7325
(603)-271-6200
(800) 322-9191

CONWAY
73 Hobbs Street
Conway, NH 03818-6188
(603) 447-3841
(800) 552-4628

KEENE
809 Court Street
Keene, NH 03431-0744
(603) 357-3510
(800) 624-9700

LACONIA
65 Beacon Street West
Laconia, NH 03247-0634
(603) 524-4485
(800) 322-2121

LITTLETON
80 North Littleton Road
Littleton, NH 03561-0260
(603) 444-6786
(800) 552-8959

MANCHESTER
361 Lincoln Street
Manchester, NH 03103-4976
(603) 668-2330
(800) 852-7493

NASHUA
19 Chestnut Street
Nashua, NH 03061-1025
(603) 883-7726
(800) 852-0632

PORTSMOUTH
30 Maplewood Avenue
Portsmouth, NH 03801-0599
(603) 433-8400
(800) 821-0326

ROCHESTER
150 Wakefield Street
Rochester, NH 03867-3193
(603) 332-9120
(800) 862-5300

SALEM
154 Main Street
Salem, NH 03079-3191
(603) 893-9763
(800) 852-7492

NEW JERSEY PUBLIC HUMAN SERVICE AGENCIES

ATLANTIC
1333 Atlantic Avenue
Atlantic City, NJ 08401
(609) 348-3001
Fax: (609) 345-4295

BERGEN
216 Route 17 North
17 Park Office Center, Building A
Rochelle Park, NJ 07662-3300
(201) 368-4200
(201) 368-8710

BURLINGTON
795 Woodlane Road
Mount Holly, NJ 08060-3316
(609) 261-1000
Fax: (609) 261-0463

CAMDEN
County Administration Building
600 Market Street
Camden, NJ 08101
(609) 225-8800
Fax: (609) 225-7797

CAPE MAY
4005 Route 9 South
Rio Grande, NJ 08242-1911
(609) 886-6200
Fax: (609) 889-9332

CUMBERLAND
13 North East Boulevard
Vineland, NJ 08360
(609) 691-4600
Fax: (609) 692-7635

ESSEX
18 Rector Street, 9th Floor
Newark, NJ 07102
(973) 733-3000
Fax: (973) 643-3985

GLOUCESTER
400 Hollydell Drive
Sewell, NJ 08080
(609) 582-9200
Fax: (609) 582-6587

HUDSON
100 Newkirk Street
Jersey City, NJ 07306
(201) 420-3000
Fax: (201) 420-0343

HUNTERDON
Community Services Center
6 Gauntt Place
Flemington, NJ 08822
(908) 788-1300
Fax: (908) 806-4569

MERCER
200 Woolverton Street
PO Box 1450
Trenton, NJ 08650-2099
(609) 989-4494
Fax: (609) 989-0405

MIDDLESEX
181 Howe Lane, PO Box 509
New Brunswick, NJ 08903
(732) 745-3500
Fax: (732) 745-4555

MONMOUTH
Kozloski Road, PO Box 3000
Freehold, NJ 07728
(908) 431-6000
Fax: (908) 431-6267

MORRIS
Mount Pleasant Complex, Lobby C
1719 Route 10
Parsippany, NJ 07054
(201) 326-7800
Fax: (201) 326-7251

OCEAN
1027 Hooper Avenue
PO Box 547
Toms River, NJ 08754-0547
(908) 349-1500
Fax: (908) 244-8075

PASSAIC
80 Hamilton Street
Paterson, NJ 07505-2057
(973) 881-0100
Fax: (973) 881-3232

SALEM
147 South Virginia Avenue
Penns Grove, NJ 08069
(609) 299-7200
Fax: (609) 299-3245

SOMERSET
73 East High Street
PO Box 936
Somerville, NJ 08876
(908) 5260-8800
Fax: (908) 231-9010

SUSSEX
18 Church Street
PO Box 218
Newton, NJ 07860-0218
(973) 383-3600
Fax: (973) 3883-3627

UNION
342 Westminster Avenue
Elizabeth, NJ 07208-3290
(908) 965-2700
Fax: (908) 965-2752

WARREN
Court House Annex
Second & Hardwick Streets
Box 3000
Belvidere, NJ 07823-3000
(908) 475-4744
Fax: (908) 475-1533

NEW MEXICO MEDICAL ASSISTANCE DIVISION

SOUTH EAST BERNALILLO
1401 Williams South East
PO Box 543
Albuqureque, NM 87103
(505) 841-2600
(800) 826-1468
Fax: (505) 841-2105

SOUTH WEST BERNALILLO
1401 Old Coors Rd South West
PO Box 12355
Albuquerque, NM 87195
(505) 841-2300
Fax: (505) 841-2381

NORTH WEST BERNALILLO
1011 Lamberton Place NE
PO Box 25287
Albuquerque, NM 87195
(505) 841-7700
Fax: (505) 841-7757

NORTH EAST BERNALILLO
1011 Lamberton Place NE
PO Box 25287
Albuquerque, NM 87125
(505) 841-7700
Fax: (505) 841-7917

CATRON-CONTACT SOCORRO COUNTY ISD

CHAVES
1701 South Sunset
Roswell, NM 88201
(505) 625-3000
(800) 824-8971
Fax: (505) 625-3099

COLFAX
1900 Hospital Drive
PO Box 368
Raton, NM 87740
(505) 445-2308
(800) 624-3469
Fax: (505) 445-2218

CURRY
1621 Suter Place
Clovis, NM 88101
(505) 762-4751
Fax: (505) 763-0493

DEBACA-CONTAACT GUADALUPE COUNTY ISD

DONA ANA
750 North Motel Boulevard, Bldg A
Las Cruces, NM 88005
(505) 524-6500
(800) 457-0631
Fax: (505) 524-6509

EDDY
2324 West Pierce Street
Carlsbad, NM 88220
(505) 885-8815
(800) 624-6926
Fax: (505) 887-0550

GRANT
1422 Highway 180 East
Silver City, NM 88061
(505) 538-2948
(800) 331-7311
Fax: (505) 538-0241

GUADALUPE
200 Lake Drive
PO Box 369
Santa Rosa, NM 88061
(505) 472-3450
(800) 523-6643
Fax: (505) 472-3425

HARDING-CONTACT SAN MIGUEL COUNTY ISD
HIDALGO-CONTACT GRANT COUNTY ISD

LEA
2120 North Alto, Suite D
Hobbs, NM 88240
(505) 397-3400
(800) 558-8270
Fax: (505) 393-2529

LINCOLN
PO Box 1400
Ruidoso, NM 88345
(505) 257-6165
Fax: (505) 257-6961

LOS ALAMOS-CONTACT RIO ARRIBA COUNTY ISD

LUNA
116 East Poplar
PO Box 818
Deming, NM 88030
(505) 546-0467
Fax: (505) 546-9326

MCKINLEY
2907 East Aztec
Gallup, NM 87301
(505) 863-9545
(800) 825-7422
Fax: (505) 722-0991

MORA-CONTACT SAN MIGUEL COUNTY ISD

OTERO
108 Cottonwood
PO Drawer E'Alamogordo, NM 88310
(505) 437-9260
(800) 826-4468
Fax: (505) 437-3098

QUAY
612 East Main Street
PO Box 868
Tucumcari, NM 88401
(505) 461-4627
(800) 548-3956
Fax: (505) 461-2983

RIO ARRIBA
Highway 84 Welfare Building
PO Box 2125
Espanola, NM 87532
(505) 753-2271
(800) 231-2835
Fax: (505) 753-5826

ROOSEVELT
1028 Community Way
PO Box 1090
Portales, NM 88130
(505) 356-4473
Fax: (505) 359-2142

SANDOVAL
830 Camino Del Pueblo
PO Box 430
Bernalillo, NM 87004
(505) 867-3357
(800) 926-9425
Fax: (505) 867-9492

SAN JUAN
101 West Animas
PO Box 5250
Farmington, NM 87499
(505) 325-1831
(800) 231-6668
Fax: (505) 599-9658

SAN MIGUEL
3112 Hot Springs Boulevard
PO Box 1348
Las Vegas, NM 87701
(505) 425-6741
Fax: (505) 454-0256

SANTA FE
2542 Cerrillos Road
Station A
Santa Fe, NM 87505
(505) 827-1900
(800) 231-8081
Fax: (505) 827-1939

SIERRA
102 Barton Street
T or C, NM 87901
(505) 894-3011
Fax: (505) 894-1021

SOCORRO
302 Park Avenue South West
PO Box LL
Socorro, NM 87801
(505) 835-0342
(800) 245-9571
Fax: (505) 835-9478

TAOS
Mary Medina Building
PO Box HH
Taos, NM 87571
(505) 758-8804
Fax: (505) 758-1012

TORRANCE
507 Williams Street
PO Box 765
Estancia, NM 87016-0765
(505) 384-3151 or (505) 384-3154
Fax: (505) 384-2528

UNION
834 Main Street
Clayton, NM 88415
(505) 374-2854
Fax: (505) 374-2853
Message: (505) 374-9401

VALENCIA
Fifth and Becker
PO Box 259
Belen, NM 87002
(505) 864-5200
Fax: (505) 864-5247

CIBOLA
900 Mt Taylor Avenue
Grants, NM 87020
(505) 287-8836
(800) 558-8270
Fax: (505) 285-6278

ARTESIA
509 West Mahone
Artesia, NM 88210
(505) 748-3361
Fax: (505) 746-6123

LOVINGTON-CONTACT LEA COUNTY ISD

SO DONA ANA
826 North Anthony Drive
PO Box 4130
Anthony, NM 88021
(505) 882-5781
Fax: (505) 882-4728

NEW YORK STATE DEPARTMENT OF SOCIAL SERVICES

ALBANY
162 Washington Avenue
Albany, NY 12207
(518) 447-7300 Reception
Fax: (518) 447-7722
(518) 447-7011 (Nursing Home)
(518) 447-7017 (Chronic Care)

ALLEGANY
7 Court Street
Belmont, NY 14813
(716) 268-9622
Fax: (716) 268-9479

BROOME
36 Main Street
Binghamton, NY 13905
(607) 772-2615

CATTARAUGUS
Olean, Main Office
1701 Lincoln Avenue, Suite 600
Olean, NY 14760-1158
(716) 373-8065

CATTARAUGUS-LITTLE VALLEY OFFICE
200 Erie Street
Little Valley, NY 14755
(716) 938-6913

CATTARAUGUS-SALAMANCA OFFICE
100 Main Street
Salamanca, NY 14779
(716) 945-2093

CAYUGA
Cayuga County Office Bldg, 2nd Floor
160 Genesee Street
Auburn, NY 13021
(315) 253-1404
Fax: (315) 253-1560

CHAUTAUQUA
H.R. Clothier Building
Mayville, NY 14757
(716) 661-8040 and (716) 661-8200

CHEMUNG
425 Pennsylvania Avenue
Elmira, NY 14902-0588
(607) 737-5360

CHENANGO
5 Court Street
PO Box 590
Norwich, NY 13815
(607) 337-1511

CLINTON
13 Durkee Street
Plattsburgh, NY 12901
(518) 565-3300

COLUMBIA
25 Railroad Avenue
PO Box 458
Hudson, NY 12534
(518) 828-9411 ask for Medicaid Department

CORTLAND
60 Central Avenue
County Office Bldg
Cortland, NY 13045
(607) 753-5303

DELAWARE
111 Main Street
Delhi, NY 13753
(607) 746-2325
Fax: (607) 746-6310

DUTCHESS
60 Market Street
Poughkeepsie, NY 12601
(845) 486-3000

ERIE
95 Franklin Street
Buffalo, NY 14202-3959
(716) 858-6582

ESSEX
Court Street
PO Box 217
Elizabethtown, NY 12932
(518) 873-3450

FRANKLIN
Court House, 2nd Floor
Malone, NY 12953
(518) 481-1808 Reception

FULTON
PO Box 549
Johnstown, NY 12095
(518) 736-5600

GENESEE
County Building II
3837 West Main Rd
Batavia, NY 14020
(716) 344-8502 ask for Medicaid

GREENE
465 Main Street
PO Box 528
Catskill, NY 12414
(518) 943-3200
Fax: (518) 943-4730

HAMILTON
White Birch Lane
PO Box 725
Indian Lake, NY 12842
(518) 648-6131
Fax: (518) 648-5257

HERKIMER
301 North Washington Street
PO Box 231
Herkimer, NY 13350
(315) 867-1291

JEFFERSON
250 Arsensal Street
Watertown, NY 13601
(315) 782-9030
Fax: (315) 785-3019

LEWIS
Outerstowe Street
PO Box 193
Lowville, NY 13367
(315) 376-5400

LIVINGSTON
3 Livingston Co. Campus
Mt. Morris, NY 14510
(716) 243-7300
Fax: (716) 243-7364

MADISON
PO Box 637
Wampsville, NY 13163
(315) 363-2479

MONROE
111 Westfall Road
Rochester, NY 14620
(716) 274-6441

MONTGOMERY
County Office Bldg (on Broadway)
PO Box 745
Fonda, NY 12068
(518) 853-4646

NASSAU
101 County Seat Drive
Mineola, NY 11501-4821
(516) 571-4558

NEW YORK CITY
Human Resources Administration (HRA)
250 Church Street, Room 1500
New York, NY 10013-3403
Automated Attendant can be reached for more details at the following numbers:
(718) 291-1900 or toll free at (877) 742-8411
Serves the boroughs of Bronx, Brooklyn, Manhattan, Queens, and Richmond (Staten Island). Note this will require a minimum of two separate appointments. First, will be the application, then the interview.

NEW YORK CITY-BRONX:

Bronx Lebanon Hospital Medicaid Office
1278 Fulton Avenue
Bronx, NY 10456
(718) 588-2997

Lincoln Hospital Medicaid Office
234 East 149th Street
Basement-Room B75)
Bronx, NY 10451
(718) 585-3224

Morrisania Medicaid Office
1225 Gerard Avenue
(Basement)
Bronx, NY 10452
(718) 960-2799

North Central Bronx Hospital Medicaid Office
3424 Kossuth Avenue
(1st Floor-Room 1A05)
Bronx, NY 10456
(718) 920-1070

St. Barnabas Hospital Medicaid Office
4422 Third Avenue (3rd Floor)
Bronx, NY 10457
(718) 960-6325

NEW YORK CITY-BROOKLYN:

Boerum Hill Medicaid Office
88 Third Avenue (1st Floor)
Brooklyn, NY 11217
(718) 694-8722 or (718) 694-8723

Bushwick Medicaid Office
737 Flushing Avenue (4th Floor)
Brooklyn, NY 11206
(718) 963-5080 or (718) 963-5081

Coney Island Medicaid Office
2865 West 8th Street (Main Floor)
Brooklyn, NY 11224
(718) 265-5601 or (718) 265-5602

Kings County Hospital Medicaid Office
441 Clarkson Avenue "T" Bldg. (1st Floor)
Brooklyn, NY 11203
(718) 221-2300 or (718) 221-2301

NEW YORK CITY-MANHATTAN:

Bellevue Hospital Medicaid Office
466 First Avenue & 27th Street "G" Link
(1st Floor)
New York, NY
(212) 679-7153 or (212) 679-7258

Gouverneur Hospital Medicaid Office
227 Madison Street (7th Floor)
New York, NY 10002
(212) 238-7790

Harlem Medicaid Office
6-20 West 137th Street (Room 130)
(The Old Pediatrics Bldg)
New York, NY 10037
(212) 281-1240

Metropolitan Hospital Medicaid Office
1901 First Avenue (1st Floor-Room 1D18)
New York, NY 10002
(212) 423-6583

Presbyterian Hospital Medicaid Office
622 West 168th Street (First Floor) PH040
New York, NY 10032
(212) 342-5102 or (212) 342-5103

NEW YORK CITY-QUEENS:

Elmhurst Hospital Medicaid Office
79-01 Broadway (Room C4-5)
Elmhurst, NY 11373
(718) 476-5904

Far Rockaway Medicaid Office
220 Beach 87th Street (Street Level)
Far Rockaway, NY 11693
(718) 318-6580 or (718) 318-6581

Jamaica Medicaid Office
90-75 Sutphin Boulevard (8th Floor)
Jamaica, NY 11453
(718) 523-6289

NEW YORK CITY-RICHMOND:

Staten Island Medicaid Office
350 St. Marks Place (Basement)
Staten Island, NY 10301
(718) 720-2850 or (718) 720-2851

NIAGARA
100 Davidson Road
PO Box 865
Lockport, NY 14095-0506
(716) 439-7777

ONEIDA
800 Park Avenue
Utica, NY 13501
(315) 798-5632

ONONDAGA
Onondaga County Civic Center
421 Montgomery Street
Syracuse, NY 13202
(315) 435-2928

ONTARIO
3010 County Complex Drive
Canandaigua, NY 14424
(716) 396-4060 and (716) 396-4061
Fax: (716) 396-4597

ONTARIO (GENEVA OFFICE)
28 Seneca Street
Geneva, NY 14456
(315) 789-2841
Fax: (315) 789-1767
Serves zip codes: 14456, 14532, and 13165

ORANGE
23 Hatfield Lane
Goshen, NY 10924
(914) 291-2800

ORANGE-GOSHEN
Box Z, Quarry Road
Goshen, NY 10924
(914) 294-4000

ORANGE-MIDDLETOWN
33 Fulton Plaza
Middletown, NY 10940
(914) 346-1120

ORANGE-NEWBURG
141 Broadway
Newburg, NY 12550
(914) 568-5100

ORANGE-PORT JERVIS
150 Pike Street
Port Jervis, NY 12771
(914) 858-1420

ORLEANS
14016 Route 31 West
Albion, NY 14411
(716) 589-7000
Fax: (716) 589-7479

OSWEGO
100 Spring Street
PO Box 1320
Mexico, NY 13114
(315) 963-5000
(888) 963-5377
Fax: (315) 963-5477

OSTEGO
197 Main Street
Cooperstown, NY 13326
(607) 544-2100

PUTNAM
110 Old Rt. 6 Center.
Carmel, NY 10512
(914) 225-7040 (Note, Automated Voice Menu. Enter 1251 for Medicaid)
Fax: (914) 225-8635

QUEENS–SEE NEW YORK CITY

RENSSELAER
133 Bloomingrove Drive
Troy, NY 12180
(518) 270-3928

ROCKLAND COUNTY DSS
Sanatorium Rd
Bldg L
Pomona, NY 10970
(914) 364-3990 (Nursing Home Unit)

SAINT LAWRENCE
Harold B. Smith Office Bldg
Judson Street
Canton, NY 13617
(315) 379-2111

SARATOGA
152 West High Street
Ballston Spa, NY 12020
(518) 884-4148

SCHENECTADY
487 Nott Street
Schenectady, NY 12308-1895
(518) 388-4470

SCHOHARIE
300 Main Street
County Office Building, 2nd Floor
PO Box 687
Schoharie, NY 12157
(518) 295-8334
Fax: (518) 295-8499

SCHUYLER
County Office Bldg
105 Ninth Street
Watkins Glen, NY 14891
(607) 535-8303

SENECA
PO Box 690
1 DiPronio Drive
Waterloo, NY 13165
(315) 539-1447

STEUBEN
3 East Pulteney Square
Bath, NY 14810
(607) 776-7611
Fax: (607) 776-7188

SUFFOLK
3085 Veterans Highway
Ronkonkoma, NY 11779
(631) 854-5866 or (631) 854-5895

SULLIVAN
Box 231
Infirmary Road
Liberty, NY 12754
(914) 292-0100 (Note, Push 5 for Operator Assistance! Ask for Nursing Home Medicaid)
Fax: (914) 292-1320

TIOGA
1062 State Rte 38
PO Box 240
Owego, NY 13827
(607) 687-8300

TOMPKINS
320 West State Street
Ithaca, NY 14850
(607) 274-5328 Information
(607) 274-5359 Appointments

ULSTER
1061 Development Court
Kingston, NY 12401-1959
(914) 334-5000

WARREN
Warren County Municipal Center
1340 State Rte 9
Lake George, NY 12845
(518) 761-6321 (Note, application mailed only. Informed of no prior screening policy)

WASHINGTON
383 Broadway
Fort Edward, NY 12828
(518) 746-2300

WAYNE
PO Box 10
77 Water Street
Lyons, NY 14489-0010
(315) 946-4881
Fax: (315) 946-6810

WESTCHESTER
112 East Post Road
White Plains, NY 10601-4201
(914) 285-5000

WYOMING
466 North Main Street
PO Box 231
Warsaw, NY 14569
(716) 786-8900

YATES
110 Court Street
Penn Yan, NY 14527
(315) 536-5183
Fax: (315) 536-5168

NORTH CAROLINA COUNTY DEPARTMENTS OF SOCIAL SERVICES

ALAMANCE
PO Box 3406
Burlington, NC 27217
(336) 570-6532
Fax: (336) 570-6499

ALEXANDER
334 7th Street, South West
Taylorsville, NC 28681-2413
(828) 632-1080
Fax: (828) 632-1092

ALLEGHANY
PO Box 247
Sparta, NC 28675
(336) 372-2411
Fax: (336) 372-2635

ANSON
118 North Washington Street
Wadesboro, NC 28170
(704) 694-9351
Fax: (704) 695-1608

ASHE
PO Box 298
Jefferson, NC 28640
(336) 246-1900
Fax: (336) 246-6231

AVENUERY
PO Box 309
Newland, NC 28657
(828) 733-8230
Fax: (828) 733-8245

BEAUFORT
PO Box 1358
Washington, NC 27889
(252) 975-5500
Fax: (252) 975-5555

BERTIE
PO Box 627
Windsor, NC 27983
(252) 794-5320
Fax: (252) 794-5344

BLADEN
PO Box 369
Elizabethtown, NC 28337
(910) 862-6800
Fax: (910) 862-6801

BRUNSWICK
PO Box 219
Bolivia, NC 28422-0219
(910) 253-2077
Fax: (910) 253-2071

BUNCOMBE
PO Box 7408
Asheville, NC 28801
(828) 250-5500
Fax: (828) 255-5845

BURKE
PO Box 549
Morganton, NC 28680-0549
(828) 439-2000
Fax: (828) 439-2137

CABARRUS
1303 South Cannon Boulevard
Kannapolis, NC 28083
(704) 939-1400
Fax: (704) 939-1401

CALDWELL
1966-H Morganton Boulevard, South West
Lenoir, NC 28645
(828) 757-1180
Fax: (828) 757-1189

CAMDEN
PO Box 70
Camden, NC 27921
(252) 331-4787
Fax: (252) 335-1009

CARTERET
PO Box 779
Beaufort, NC 28516
(252) 728-3181
Fax: (252) 728-3631

CASWELL
Drawer S
Yanceyville, NC 27379
(336) 694-4141
Fax: (336) 694-1816

CATAWBA
PO Box 669
Newton, NC 28658
(828) 326-5600
Fax: (828) 322-2497

CHATHAM
PO Box 489
Pittsboro, NC 27312
(919) 542-2759
Fax: (919) 542-6355

CHEROKEE
40 Peachtree Street
Murphy, NC 28906
(828) 837-7455
Fax: (828) 837-9789

CHOWAN
PO Box 296
Edenton, NC 27932
(252) 482-7441
Fax: (252) 482-7041

CLAY
PO Box 147
Hayesville, NC 28904
(828) 389-6301
Fax: (828) 389-6427

CLEVELAND
Drawer 9006
Shelby, NC 28150-9006
(704) 487-0661
Fax: (704) 484-1051

COLUMBUS
PO Box 397
Whiteville, NC 28472-0397
(910) 642-2800
Fax: (910) 641-3970

CRAVENUEN
2818 Neuse Boulevard
PO Box 12039
New Bern, NC 28561-2039
(252) 636-4900
Fax: (252) 636-4946

CUMBERLAND
PO Box 2429
Fayetteville, NC 28302
(910) 323-1540
Fax: (910) 323-1509

CURRITUCK
PO Box 99
Currituck, NC 27929
(252) 232-3083
Fax: (252) 232-2167

DARE
PO Box 669
Manteo, NC 27954
(252) 473-1471
Fax: (252) 473-9824

DAVIDSON
PO Box 788
Lexington, NC 27292
(336) 242-2500
Fax: (336) 249-1924

DAVIE
PO Box 517
Mocksvile, NC 27028
(336) 751-8800
Fax: (336) 751-1639

DUPLIN
PO Box 969
Kenansville, NC 28349
(910) 296-2200
Fax: (910) 296-2323

DURHAM
PO Box 810
Durham, NC 27702
(919) 560-8000
Fax: (919) 560-8102

EDGECOMBE
3003 North Main Street
Tarboro, NC 27886
(252) 641-7611
Fax: (252) 641-7980

EDGECOMBE (ROCKY MOUNT OFFICE)
301 North Fairview Road
Rockymount, NC 27801
(252) 985-4101
Fax: (252) 985-1615

FORSYTH
PO Box 999
Winston-Salem, NC 27102
(336) 727-2248
Fax: (336) 727-2850

FRANKLIN
PO Box 669
Louisburg, NC 27549
(919) 496-5721
Fax: (919) 496-8137

GASTON
330 North Marietta Street
Gastonia, NC 28052
(704) 862-7500
Fax: (704) 862-7885

GATES
PO Box 185
Gatesville, NC 27938
(252) 357-0075
Fax: (252) 357-2132

GRAHAM
PO Box 1150
Robbinsville, NC 28771
(828) 479-7911
Fax: (828) 479-7928

GRANVILLE
PO Box 966
Oxford, NC 27565
(919) 693-1511
Fax: (919) 603-5090

GREENE
227 Kingold Boulevard, Suite A
Snow Hill, NC 28580
(252) 747-5932
Fax: (252) 747-8654

GUILFORD
PO Box 3388
Greensboro, NC 27402
(336) 373-3813
Fax: (336) 333-6868

HALIF
PO Box 767
Halif, NC 27839
(252) 536-2511
Fax: (252) 536-6539

HARNETT
311 Cornelius Harnett Boulevard
Lillington, NC 27546
(910) 893-7500
Fax: (910) 893-6604

HAYWOOD
486 East Marshall Street
Waynesville, NC 28786
(828) 452-6620
Fax: (828) 452-6673

HENDERSON
246 Second Avenue, East
Henderson, NC 38792
(828) 697-5500
Fax: (828) 697-4544

HERTFORD
PO Box 218
Winton, NC 27986
(252) 358-7830
Fax: (252) 358-0597

HOKE
PO Box 340
Raeford, NC 28376
(910) 875-8725
Fax: (910) 875-1068

HYDE
PO Box 220
Swan Quarter, NC 27885
(252) 926-3371
Fax: (252) 926-3081

IREDELL
PO Box 1146
Statesville, NC 28677
(704) 873-5631
Fax: (704) 878-5419

JACKSON
538 Scotts Creek Road, Suite 200
Sylva, NC 28779
(828) 586-5546
Fax: (828) 586-6270

JOHNSTON
PO Box 911
Smithfield, NC 27577
(919) 989-5300
Fax: (919) 989-5324

JONES
PO Box 250
Trenton, NC 28585
(252) 448-2581
Fax: (252) 448-5651

LEE
PO Box 1066
Sanford, NC 27331-1066
(919) 718-4690
Fax: (919) 718-4634

LENOIR
PO Box 6
Kinston, NC 28502-0006
(252) 559-6400
Fax: (252) 559-6380

LINCOLN
PO Box 130
Lincolnton, NC 28093-0130
(704) 732-0738
Fax: (704) 736-8692

MACON
5 West Main Street
Franklin, NC 28734
(828) 349-2124
Fax: (828) 524-1071

MADISON
PO Box 219
Marshall, NC 28753
(828) 649-2711
Fax: (828) 649-2097

MARTIN
PO Box 809
Williamston, NC 27892
(252) 809-6400
Fax: (252) 792-5186

MCDOWELL
PO Box 338
Marion, NC 28752
(828) 652-3355
Fax: (828) 652-9167

MECKLENBURG
301 Billingsley Road
Charlotte, NC 28211
(704) 336-3150
Fax: (704) 336-3361

MITCHELL
PO Box 365
Bakersville, NC 28705-0365
(828) 688-2175
Fax: (828) 688-4940

MONTGOMERY
PO Drawer N
Troy, NC 27371
(910) 576-6531
Fax: (910) 576-5016

MOORE
PO Box 938
Carthage, NC 28327
(910) 947-2436
Fax: (910) 947-1618

NASH
PO Drawer 819
Nashville, NC 27856
(252) 459-9818
Fax: (252) 459-9833

NEW HANOVER
1650 Greenfield Street
Wilmington, NC 28401
(910) 341-4700
Fax: (910) 341-4022

NORTH AMPTON
PO Box 157
Jackson, NC 27845
(252) 534-5811
Fax: (252) 534-0061

ONSLOW
PO Box 1379
Jacksonville, NC 28541-1379
(910) 455-4145
Fax: (910) 455-2901

ORANGE
300 West Tryon Street
Hillsborough, NC 27278
(919) 732-9361
Fax: (919) 644-33005

PAMLICO
PO Box 395
Bayboro, NC 28515
(252) 745-4086
Fax: (252) 745-7384

PASQUOTANK
709 Roanoke Avenue
Elizabeth City, NC 27907
(252) 338-2126
Fax: (252) 338-7512

PENDER
PO Box 1207
Burgaw, NC 28425
(910) 259-1240
Fax: (910) 259-1418

PERQUIMANS
PO Box 107
Hertford, NC 27944
(252) 426-7373
Fax: (252) 426-1788

PERSON
PO Box 770
Roxboro, NC 27573
(336) 599-8361
Fax: (336) 597-9339

PITT
1717 West Fifth Street
Greenville, NC 27834-1695
(252) 413-1101
Fax: (252) 413-1252

POLK
500 Carolina Drive
Tryon, NC 28782
(828) 859-5825
Fax: (828) 589-9703

RANDOLPH
PO Box 3239
Asheboro, NC 27204-3239
(336) 683-8000
Fax: (336) 683-8131

RICHMOND
PO Box 518
Rockingham, NC 28379
(910) 997-8400
Fax: (910) 997-8447

ROBESON
435 Caton Road
Lumberton, NC 28360
(910) 671-3500
Fax: (910) 671-3092

ROCKINGHAM
PO Box 361
Wentworth, NC 27375
(336) 342-1394
Fax: (336) 634-1847

ROWAN
1236 West Innes Street
Salisbury, NC 28144
(704) 633-4921
Fax: (704) 638-3041

RUTHERFORD
PO Box 237
Spindale, NC 28160
(828) 287-6199
Fax: (828) 287-6350

SAMPSON
PO Box 1105
Clinton, NC 28329
(910) 592-7131
Fax: (910) 592-4297

SCOTLAND
PO Box 1647
Laurinburg, NC 28353
(910) 277-2525
Fax: (910) 277-2402

STANLY
1000 North First Street, Suite 2
Albemarle, NC 28001
(704) 982-6100
Fax: (704) 983-5818

STOKES
PO Box 30
Danbury, NC 27016
(336) 593-2861
Fax: (336) 593-9362

SURRY
118 Hamby Road
Dobson, NC 27017
(336) 401-8700
Fax: (336) 401-8750

SWAIN
PO Drawer 610
Bryson City, NC 28713
(828) 488-6921
Fax: (828) 488-2754

TRANSYLVANIA
207 South Broad Street
Brevard, NC 28712
(828) 884-3174
Fax: (828) 884-3263

TYRRELL
PO Box 449
Columbia, NC 27925
(252) 796-3421
Fax: (252) 796-1732

UNION
1212 West Roosevelt Boulevard
Monroe, NC 28111-0489
(704) 296-4300
Fax: (704) 296-6151

VANCE
350 Ruin Creek Road
Henderson, NC 27536
(252) 492-5001
Fax: (252) 438-5977

WAKE
PO Box 46833
Raleigh, NC 27620
(919) 212-7000
Fax: (919) 212-7027

WARREN
307 North Main Street
Warrenton, NC 27580
(252) 257-5000
Fax: (252) 257-4656

WASHINGTON
PO Box 10
Plymouth, NC 27962
(252) 793-4041
Fax: (252) 793-3195

WATAUGA
132 Poplar Grove Road Connector, Suite C
Boone, NC 28607
(828) 265-8100
Fax: (828) 265-7638

WAYNE
301 North Herman Street, Box HH
Goldsboro, NC 27530
(919) 731-1048
Fax: (919) 731-1350

WILKES
PO Box 119
Wilkesboro, NC 28697
(336) 651-7400
Fax: (336) 651-7568

WILSON
PO Box 459
Wilson, NC 27894-0459
(252) 206-4000
Fax: (252) 237-1544

YADKIN
PO Box 548
Yadkinville, NC 27055
(336) 679-4210
Fax: (336) 679-2664

YANCEY
PO Box 67
Burnsville, NC 28714
(828) 682-6148 or (828) 682-2470
Fax: (828) 682-6712

NORTH DAKOTA

Directory County Social Service Boards

ADAMS
606 2nd Avenue North
Hettinger, ND 58639
Mail to: PO Box 550
Hettinger, ND 58639
(701) 567-2967
Fax: (701) 567-2910

BARNES
230 4th St NW Rm. 105
Valley City, ND 58072-2994
(701) 845-8521
Fax: (701) 845-4281

BENSON
130 Main Street East
Minnewaukan, ND 58351-0186
Mail to: PO Box 186
Minnewaukan, ND 583351-0186
(701) 473-5302
Fax: (701) 473-2511
TTY 701-662-7088

BILLINGS
70 SE 1st Street
Beach, ND 58621-0279
Mail to: PO Box 279
Beach, ND 58621-0279
(701) 872-4121 or (701) 872-4122
Fax: (701) 872-3141

BOTTINEAU
314 5th Street West, Suite 1
Bottineeau, ND 58313
(701) 228-3613
Fax: (701) 228-2336

BOWMAN
104 West 1st
PO Box 269
Bowman, ND 58623
(701) 523-3285
Fax: (701) 523-3428

BURKE
103 Main Street SE
PO Box 220
Bowbells, ND 58721
(701) 377-2313
Fax: (701) 377-2302
TTY (701) 377-2318

BURLEIGH
415 E Rosser Avenue, Suite 113
Bismark, ND 58501-4058
(701) 222-6622
Fax: (701) 222-6644
TTY (701) 222-6622

CASS
1010 2nd Avenue South
PO Box 2986
Fargo, ND 58108-2988
(701) 241-5781
Fax: (701) 239-6820
TTY (701) 239-6784

CAVALIER
324 7th Avenue
PO Box 630
Langdon, ND 58249
(701) 256-2175
Fax: (701) 256-2179
TTY (701) 256-2311

DICKEY
Highway 281 North
PO Box 279
Ellendale, ND 58436
(701) 349-3271
Fax: (701) 349-3277

DIVIDE
300 2nd Avenue N
PO Box 9
Crosby, ND 58730-0009
(701) 965-6521
Fax: (701) 965-6943

DUNN
215 Central Street
Killdear, ND 58640
(701) 764-5385
Fax: (701) 764-5070

EDDY
22 9th Street South
New Rockford, ND 58356
(701) 947-5314
Fax: (701) 947-2960
TTY (701) 947-5003

EMMONS
100 NW 4th Avenue
PO Box 726
Linton, ND 58552
(701) 254-4502
Fax: (701) 254-4012

FOSTER
1000 North Central Avenue
PO Box 80
Carrington, ND 58421
(701) 652-2221
(701) 652-2173

GOLDEN VALLEY
70 Se 1st Street
PO Box 279
Beach, ND 58621-0279
(701) 872-4121 or (701) 872-4122

GRAND FORKS
221 South 4th Street
Grand Forks, ND 58201-4737
(701) 772-8171
Fax: (701) 772-1428

GRANT
106 2nd Avenue NE
PO Box 278
Carson, ND 58529
(701) 622-3706
(701) 622-3717

GRIGGS
808 Rolling Avenue SW
PO Box 567
Cooperstown, ND 58425
(701) 797-2127
Fax: (701) 797-2172

HETTINGER
309 Millionaire Avenue
PO Box 228
Mott, ND 58646
(701) 824-3276
Fax: (701) 824-2717
TTY (701) 824-2820

KIDDER
120 East Broadway
PO Box 38
Steele, ND 584482
(701) 475-2551
Fax: (701) 475-2298
TTY (701) 475-2551

LA MOURE
202 4th Avenue NE
PO Box 38
La Moure, ND 58458
(701) 883-44282
Fax: (701) 883-4244

LOGAN
318 Main
PO Box 26
Napoleon, ND 58561
(701) 754-2283
Fax: (701) 754-2282
TTY (701) 754-2283

MC HENRY
407 South Main
PO Box 58
Towner, ND 58788
(701) 537-5944
Fax: (701) 537-5417

MCINTOSH
112 NE 1st Street
PO Box 218
Ashley, ND 58413
(701)288-3343
Fax: (701) 288-3671
TTY (701) 288-3724

MCKENZIE
201 West 5th
PO Box 790
Watford City, ND 58854
(701) 842-3661
Fax: (701) 842-6436

MCLEAN
712 5th Avenue
PO Box 70
Washburn, ND 58577
(701) 462-3235
Fax: (701) 462-8131

MERCER
1030 Arthur Street
PO Box 70
Stanton, ND 58571
(701) 745-3384
Fax: (701) 745-3390

MORTON
200 2nd Avenue NW
Mandan, ND 58554-3124
(701) 787-3395
Fax: (701) 667-3384
TTY (701) 667-3380

MOUNTRAIL
Memorial Bldg 18 2nd Avenue
PO Box 39
Stanley, ND 58784-0039
(710) 628-2926
Fax: (710) 628-3175

NELSON
210 West B Avenue
PO Box 587
Lakota, ND 58344
(710) 247-2945
Fax: (710) 247-2412

OLIVER
315 Main Street
Center, ND 58530
Mail to: PO Box 145
Center, ND 58530
(710) 794-3212
Fax: (710) 794-3476

PEMBINA
300 Boundary Rd W #3
Cavalier, ND 58220
(710) 265-8441
Fax: (710) 265-8058

PIERCE
820 South Main Avenue
Rugby, ND 58368
(710) 776-5818
Fax: (710) 776-2516
TTY (710) 776-5818

RAMSEY
524 4th Avenue
PO Box 665
Devils Lake, ND 58301-0665
(710) 662-7050
Fax: (710) 662-7095
TTY (710) 662-7088

RANSOM
205 4th Avenue West
PO Box 628
Lisbon, ND 58054-0628
(710) 683-5661
Fax: (710) 683-4491

RENVILLE
217 Main Street East
PO Box 305
Mohall, ND 58761-0305
(710) 756-6374
Fax: (710) 756-7158
TTY (701) 756-6386

RICHLAND
413 3rd Avenue N, Office 6
Wahpeton, ND 58075
(701) 642-7751
Fax: (701) 642-7828
TTY (701) 642-7778

ROLETTE
212 2nd Avenue North East
PO Box 519
Rolla, ND 58367
(701) 477-3141
Fax: (701) 477-6298
TTY (701) 477-8711

SARGENT
355 Main Street
Forman, ND 58032-0156
Main to: PO Box 156
Forman, ND 58032-0156
(701) 724-3291
Fax: (701) 724-6244
TTY (701) 724-3302

SHERIDAN
215 East 2nd Street
McClusky, ND 58463
Mail to: PO Box 696
McClusky, ND 58463
(701) 363-2281
Fax: (701) 363-2702

SIOUX
302 2nd Avenue
Fort Yates, ND 58538
Mail to: PO Box B
Fort Yates, ND 58538
(710) 854-3821
Fax: (710) 854-3854

SLOPE
104 West 1st Street
Bowman, ND 58623
Mail to: PO Box 469
Bowman, ND 58623
(701) 523-3285
Fax: (701) 523-5443

STARK
664 12th Street West
Dickinson, ND 58601
(701) 264-7676
Fax: (701) 264-7315
TTY (701) 264-7675

STEELE
Washington Avenue
Finley, ND 58230
(701) 524-2584
Fax: (701) 524-1103
TTY (701) 524-2060

STUTSMAN
116 1st Street East
Jamestown, ND 58402-0809
(701) 252-7172
Fax: (701) 252-1561
TTY (701) 252-7172

TOWNER
2nd Street & 4th Avenue
Canda, ND 58324
Mail to: PO Box 604
Cando, ND 58324
(701) 968-4355
Fax: (701) 968-4342

TRAILL
West Caledonia Avenue
Hillsboro, ND 58045
Mail to: PO Box 190
Hillsboro, ND 58045
(701) 436-5220
Fax: (701) 436-5221

WALSH
701 West 6th Street
Grafton, ND 58237-1399
Fax: (701) 352-4488
TTY (701) 352-4526

WARD
400 22nd Avenue NW
Minot, ND 58702-2209
Mail to: PO Box 2209
Minot, ND 58702-2209
(701) 852-3552
Fax: (701) 857-0756
TTY (701) 875-0732

WELLS
101 North Railroad
Fressenden, ND 58438
Mail to: PO Box 266
Fressenden, ND 58438
(701) 547-3694
Fax: (701) 547-3348
TTY (701) 547-3694

WILLIAMS
316 2nd Avenue West
Williston, ND 58802
Mail to: PO Box 1569
Williston, ND 58802
(701) 572-4575
Fax: (701) 572-9794

NORTHERN MARIANA ISLANDS

We experienced difficulty in obtaining information. Please contact the following for details concerning Medicaid eligibility guidelines in the Northern Mariana Islands. The following information is available from the Health Care Financing Administration, Medicaid Officials Website.

Governor:
Honorable Froilan C. Tenorio
Commonwealth of the Northern Mariana Islands
Capitol Hill
Saipan, MP 96950
670-322-5091

Single State Agency Director:
Mr. Joseph K. P. Villagomez
Secretary for Health
Department of Public Health
Commonwealth of the Northern Mariana Islands
P.O. Box 409 CK
Saipan, MP 96950
670-234-6225

Medicaid Director:
Ms. Maria A. V. Leon Guerrero
Medical Administrator
Department of Public Health and Environmental Services
Commonwealth of the Northern Mariana Islands
P.O. Box 409 CK
Saipan, MP 96950
(670) 234-8931

OHIO DEPARTMENT OF HUMAN SERVICES

ADAMS
482 Rice Drive
West Union, OH 45693-0386
(937) 544-2371
Fax: (937) 544-5406
TTY (800) 750-0750 ext 269

ALLEN
550 West Elm Street
Lima, OH 45802-4506
Mail to: PO Box 4506
Lima, OH 45802-4506
(419) 228-2621
Fax: (419) 227-2448

ASHLAND
15 West Fourth Street
Ashland, OH 44805-2137
(419) 289-8141
Fax: (419) 281-7528

ASHTABULA
2924 Donahoe Drive
Ashtabula, OH 44004-4596
(440) 998-1110
Fax: (440) 998-1538

ATHENS
184 North Lancaster Street
Athens, OH 45701-1699
(740) 592-4477 and (740) 592-4479
(800) 762-3775 and (800) 338-4484
Fax: (740) 797-2447

AUGLAIZE
12 North Wood Street
Wapakoneta, OH 45895-0368
Mail to: PO Box 368
Wapakoneta, OH 45895-0368
(419) 738-4311
Fax: (419) 738-5544

BELMONT
310 Fox Shannon Place
Street Clairsville, OH 43950-9765
(740) 695-1074
Fax: (740) 695-9145

BROWN
775 Mt. Orab Pike
Georgetown, OH 45121-1399
Mail to: PO Box 169
Georgetown, OH 45121-1399
(937) 378-6104
Fax: ((37) 378-4753

BUTLER
860 North West Washington Boulevard
Hamilton, OH 45013
(513) 887-4000
Fax: (513) 887-4296 and (513) 887-4334
TTY/TDD (513) 887-4322

CARROLL
95 East Main Street
Carrollton, OH 44615-0216
Mail to: PO Box 216
Carrollton, OH 44615-0216
(330) 627-2571
Fax: (330) 627-3904

CHAMPAIGN
1512 South US Highway 68, Suite N100
Urbana, OH 43078-9288
(937) 652-1346
Fax: (937) 652-1145

CLARK
1345 Lagonda Avenue
Springfield, OH 45503-4401
(937) 327-1700
Fax: (937) 327-1996
TTY/TDD (937) 327-1873

CLERMONT
2400 Clermont Center Drive, Suite 106D
Batavia, OH 45103-2710
(513) 732-7111
Fax: (513) 732-7216

CLINTON
180 East Sugartree Street
Wilmington, OH 45177-0568
Mail to: PO Box 631
Wilmington, OH 45177-0568
(937) 382-0963
Fax: (937) 382-7039

COLUMBIANA
110 Nelson Avenue
Lisbon, OH 44432
(330) 424-1471
Fax: (330) 424-1455
TTY/TDD (330) 424-7767

COSHOCTON
725 Pine Street
Coshocton, OH 43812-0098
(740) 622-1020
Fax: (740) 622-5591

CRAWFORD
224 Norton Way
Bucyus, OH 44820-1831
(419) 562-0015
Fax: (419) 562-1056

CUYAHOGA
1219 Ontario Street, Room 424
Cleveland, OH 44114-2900
Mail to: 1641 Payne Avenue, Room 520
Cleveland, OH 44114-2900
(216) 987-6640
Fax: (216) 443-5884
TTY (216) 987-8297

DARKE
365 Martin Street
Greenville, OH 45331-0869
Mail to: PO Box 869
Greenville, OH 45331-0869
(937) 548-3840
Fax: (937) 548-8723

DEFIANCE
618 Clinton Street
Defiance, OH 443512-0639
Mail to: PO Box 639
Defiance, OH 43512-0639
(419) 782-3881 and (800) 342-0160
Fax: (419) 784-3249

DELAWARE
149 North Sandusky Street
Delaware, OH 43015-1789
(740) 368-1990
Fax: (740) 368-1989

ERIE
221 West Parish Street
Sandusky, OH 44870-4886
(419) 626-6781
Fax: (419) 626-5854
TTY/TDD (419) 626-6781

FAIRFIELD
121 East Chestnut Street
Lancaster, OH 43130-0890
Mail to: PO Box 890
Lancaster, OH 43130-0890
(740) 653-1701 and (800) 450-8845
Fax: (740) 687-6810

FAYETTE
425 West Temple
Washington Court House, OH 43160-0220
Mail to: PO Box 220
Washington Court House, OH 43160-0220
(740) 335-0350 and (800) 845-3272
Fax: (740) 333-3571

FRANKLIN
80 East Fulton Street
Columbus, OH 43215-5127
(614) 462-5127
Fax: (614) 462-4000
TTY/TDD (614) 462-7697

FULTON
604 South Shoop Avenue, Suite 200
Wauseon, OH 43567-1731
(419) 337-0010
Fax: (419) 337-0061
TTY/TDD (419) 337-7630

GALLIA
848 Third Avenue
Gallipolis, OH 45631-1661
(740) 446-3222, ext 11
Fax: (740) 446-8942

GEAUGA
12480 Ravenwood Drive
Chardon, OH 44024-9009
Mail to: PO Box 309
Chardon, OH 44024-9009
(440) 285-9141
Fax: (440) 286-6654
TTY/TDD (440) 285-9141

GREENE
541 Ledbetter Road
Xenia, OH 45385-3699
(937) 376-2951 and (937) 376-426-8334
Fax: (937) 376-5377

GUERNSEY
324 Highland Avenue
Cambridge, OH 43725-0730
Mail to: PO Box 730
Cambridge, OH 43725-0730
(720) 432-2381 and (800) 307-8422
Fax: (740) 439-5555

HAMILTON
222 East Central Parkway
Cincinnati, OH 45202-1225
(513) 946-1000
Fax: (513) 946-2248
TTY/TDD (513) 946-1295

HANCOCK
7814 County Road 140
Findlay, OH 45839-0270
Mail to: PO Box 270
Findlay, OH 45839-0270
(419) 422-0182
Fax: (419) 422-1081

HARDIN
175 West Franklin Street, Suite 150
Kenton, OH 43326-9902
(419) 675-1130 and (800) 442-7346
Fax: (419) 675-1100

HARRISON
520 North Main Street
Cadiz, OH 43907-0239
Mail to: PO Box 239
Cadiz, OH 43907-0239
(740) 942-2171
Fax: (740) 942-2370

HENRY
104 East Washington Street-Hahn Center
Napoleon, OH 43545-0527
Mail to: PO Box 527
Napoleon, OH 43545-0527
(419) 592-0946
Fax: (419) 592-0946

HIGHLAND
1575 North High Street, Suite 100
Hillsboro, OH 45133-9442
(937) 393-4278
Fax: (937) 393-4461

HOCKING
350 State Route 664 North
Logan, OH 43138-0548
Mail to: PO Box 548
Logan, OH 43138-0548
(740) 385-5663 and (800) 599-6935
Fax: (740) 385-1911

HOLMES
85 North Grant Street
Millersburg, OH 44654-0072
Mail to: PO Box 72
Millersburg, OH 44654-0072
(330) 674-1111
Fax: (330) 674-0770

HURON
185 Shady Lane Drive
Norwalk, OH 44857-2388
(419) 668-8126 and (800) 668-5175
Fax: (419) 668-4738
TTY/TDD: (419) 668-8126

JACKSON
135 Huron Street
Jackson, OH 45640-0232
Mail to: PO Box 232
Jackson, OH 45640-0232
(740) 286-4181
Fax: (740) 286-4775
TTY/TDD (740) 286-5246

JEFFERSON
125 South Fifth Street
Steubenville, OH 43952-2885
(740) 282-0961
Fax: (740) 282-7425

KNOX
117 East High Street
Mount Vernon, OH 43050-3400
(740) 397-7177
Fax: (740) 392-8882 and (740) 392-1249

LAKE
177 Main Street
Painesville, OH 44077-9967
(440) 350-4000
Fax: (440) 350-4399
TTY/TDD (440) 350-3321

LAWRENCE
1100 South Seventh Street
Ironton, OH 45638-0539
Mail to: PO Box 539
Ironton, OH 45638-0539
(740) 532-3324
Fax: (740) 532-9490

LICKING
74 South Second Street
Newark, OH 43058-0338
Mail to: PO Box 338
Newark, OH 43058-0338
(740) 349-6575 and (800) 513-1128
Fax: (740) 349-6582

LOGAN
211 East Columbus Avenue
Bellefontaine, OH 43311-9935
(937) 599-5165
Fax: (937) 592-4395

LORAIN
42485 North Ridge Road
Elyria, OH 44035-1057
(440) 323-5726
Fax: (440) 323-6229
TTY/TDD (440) 284-4125

LUCAS
3210 Monroe Street
Caller No. 10007
Toledo, OH 43699-0007
(419) 213-8999
Fax: (419) 213-8820
TTY/TDD (419) 213-8499

MADISON
200 Midway Street
London, OH 43140-1356
(740) 852-4770 and (800) 852-0243
Fax: (740) 852-4756
TTY/TDD (740) 852-4770 and (800) 852-0243

MAHONING
709 North Garland
Youngstown, OH 44501-0600
Mail to: PO Box 600
Youngstown, OH 44501-0600
(330) 740-2600
Fax: (330) 740-2617
TTY/TDD (330) 740-2610

MARION
363 West Fairground Street
Marion, OH 43301-1817
Mail to: PO Box 1817
Marion, OH 43301-1817
(740) 387-8560
Fax: (740) 387-387-2175

MEDINA
980 North Court Street
Medina, OH 44258-1239
Mail to: PO Box 1239
Medina, OH 44258-1239
(330) 722-9283
Fax: (330) 722-9352

MEIGS
175 Race Street
Middleport, OH 45760-0191
(740) 992-2117 ext 304
Fax: (740) 992-7500
TTY/TDD (740) 992-2117

MERCER
311 South Main Street
Celina, OH 45822
(419) 586-5106
Fax: (419) 586-5643

MIAMI
2040 North County Road 25-A
Troy, OH 45373-1310
(937) 335-7142
Fax: (937) 335-2225

MONROE
100 Home Avenue
Woodsfield, OH 43793-0638
Mail to: PO Box 638
Woodsfield, OH 43793-0638
(740) 472-1602
Fax: (740) 472-5666

MONTGOMERY
14 West Fourth Street
Dayton, OH 45422-3600
Mail to: PO Box 972
Dayton, OH 45422-3600
(937) 225-6347
Fax: (937) 225-5087
TTY/TDD (937) 225-5042

MORGAN
65 West Union Avenue
McConnelsville, OH 43756-1299
(740) 962-4616 and (888) 257-9159
Fax: (740) 962-5344

MORROW
27 West High Street
Mount Gilead, OH 43338-1298
(419) 947-9111 and (800) 668-6458
Fax: (419) 947-9115

MUSKINGUM
205 North Seventh Street
Zanesville, OH 43702-0157
Mail to: PO Box 9
Zanesville, OH 43702-0157

NOBLE
38 Olive Street
Caldwell, OH 43724-0250
Mail to: PO Box 250
Caldwell, Oh 43724-0250
(740) 732-2392 and (800) 905-2732
Fax: (740) 732-4108

OTTAWA
8444 West State Route 163
Oak Harbor, OH 43449-9769
(419) 898-3688
Fax: (419) 898-2436
TTY/TDD (419) 898-3688

PAULDING
303 West Harrison Street
Paulding, OH 45879-1497
(419) 399-3756
Fax: (419) 399-4674

PERRY
212 South Main Street
New Lexington, OH 43764-0311
Mail to: PO Box 311
New Lexington, OH 43764-0311
(740) 342-3551
Fax: (740) 342-5491
TTY/TDD (740) 342-3551

PICKAWAY
110 Island Road
Circleville, OH 43113-0439
(740) 474-7588
Fax: (740) 474-9333
TTY/TDD (740) 474-7588 and (740) 474-3105

PIKE
219 West Emmitt Avenue
Waverly, OH 45690-1097
(740) 947-2171
Fax: (740) 947-7628
TTY/TDD (740) 947-5380

PORTAGE
449 South Meridian Street, Second Floor
Ravenna, OH 44266-1208
(330) 297-3750
Fax: (330) 297-3847

PREBLE
1234 Eaton-Gettysburg Road
Eaton, OH 45320-0088
(937) 456-6205
Fax: (937) 456-5591

PUTNAM
1225 East Third Street
Ottawa, OH 45875-2062
(419) 523-4580
Fax: (419) 523-6130

RICHLAND
171 Park Avenue East
Mansfield, OH 44901-9978
Mail to: PO Box 188
Mansfield, OH 44901-9978
(419) 774-5400
Fax: (419) 526-4802
TTY/TDD (419) 774-5415

ROSS
150 East Second Street
Chillicothe, OH 45601-2500
(740) 773-2651 and (800) 413-3140
Fax: (740) 773-3750
TTY/TDD (800) 750-0750

SANDUSKY
2511 Countryside Drive
Fremont, OH 43420-8968
(419) 334-3891
Fax: (419) 332-2156
TTY/TDD (419) 334-8231

SCIOTO
710 Court Street
Portsmouth, OH 45662-1347
Mail to: PO Box 1347
Portsmouth, OH 45662-1347
(740) 354-6661
Fax: (740) 353-2576

SENECA
3362 South Township Road 151
Tiffin, OH 44883-9499
(419) 447-5011 and (800) 825-5011
Fax: (419) 447-5345

SHELBY
129 East Court Street
Sidney, OH 45365-3060
(937) 498-4981
Fax: (937) 498-7396

STARK
220 East Tuscarawas Street
Canton, OH 44702-1293
(330) 452-4661
Fax: (330) 438-8928
TTY/TDD (330) 438-8879

SUMMIT
47 North Main Street
Akron, OH 44308-1991
(330) 643-8200
Fax: (330) 643-7351
TTY/TDD (330) 643-8754

TRUMBULL
106 High Street North West
Warren, OH 44482-1350
(330) 675-2000
Fax: (330) 399-7824
TTY/TDD (330) 545-4371

TUSCARAWAS
247 Stonecreek Road North West
New Philadelphia, OH 44663-6902
(330) 339-7791 and (800) 431—2347
Fax: (330) 339-6388

UNION
169 Grove Street
Marysville, OH 43040-0389
Mail to: PO Box 389
Marysville, OH 43040-0389
(937) 644-1010, (800) 248-2347 and (937) 644-1854
Fax: (937) 644-8700
TTY/TDD (937) 644-1010

VAN WERT
114 East Main Street
Van Wert, OH 45891-0595
Mail to: PO Box 595
Van Wert, OH 45891-0595
(419) 238-5430
Fax: (419) 238-6045

VINTON
123 East Main Street
McArthur, OH 45651-1295
(740) 596-2581, (740) 596-4310 and (800) 482-2920
Fax: (740) 596-4562

WARREN
416 South East Street
Lebanon, OH 45036-2314
(513) 695-1420
Fax: (513) 695-2940

WASHINGTON
1115 Gilman Avenue
Marietta, OH 45750-0975
Mail to: PO Box 2005
Marietta, OH 45750-0975
(740) 373-5513
Fax: (740) 374-7692
TTY/TDD (740) 373-5513

WAYNE
356 West North Street
Wooster, OH 44691-0076
Mail to: PO Box 76
Wooster, OH 44691-0076
(330) 287-5800
Fax: (330) 287-5899

WILLIAMS
117 West Butler Street
Bryan, OH 43506-1650
(419) 636-6725
Fax: (419) 636-8843

WOOD
1928 East Gypsy Lane Road
Bowling Green, OH 43402-9396
Mail to: PO Box 679
Bowling Green, OH 43402-9396
(419) 352-7566
Fax: (419) 353-6091

WYANDOT
137 South Sandusky Avenue
Upper Sandusky, OH 43351-0510
Mail to: PO Box 510
Upper Sandusky, OH 43351-0510
(419) 294-4977
Fax: (419) 294-3501

OKLAHOMA DEPARTMENT OF HUMAN SERVICES

COUNTY OFFICES

ADAIR
Section Line Road
Rt. 1, Box 42
Stilwell, OK 74960
(918) 696-7736
(800) 225-0049
Fax: (918) 696-5419

ALFALFA
101 South Grand
PO Box 724
Cherokee, OK 73728
(580) 596-3335
(800) 225-0079
Fax: (580) 596-2414

ATOKA
PO Box 418
401 North Greathouse Drive
Atoka, OK 74525
(580) 889-3394
(800) 225-0051
Fax: (580) 889-3451

BEAVENUER
PO Box 306
111 West 2nd Street
Beaver, OK 73939
(580) 625-3441
(800) 225-0092
Fax: (580) 625-4921

BECKHAM
312 East Madden
Sayre, OK 73662
(580) 928-3348
(800) 225-0098
Fax: (580) 928-2842

BLAINE
216 West A Street
Watonga, OK 73772
(580) 623-5282
(800) 808-8961
Fax: (580) 623-5297

BRYAN
PO Box 837
4302 Highway 70 West
Durant, OK 74702
(580) 924-1866
(800) 225-0062
Fax: (580) 924-7176

CADDO
PO Box 549
201 Hardee's
Anadarko, OK 73005
405) 247-4000
(800) 225-0053
Fax: (405) 247-4025

CANADIAN
314 West Rogers Street
El Reno, OK 73036
(405) 262-2030
(800) 572-6845
Fax: (405) 262-4619

CARTER
925 West Broadway
Ardmore, OK 73401
(580) 223-6920
(800) 225-9927
Fax: (580) 223-7170

CHEROKEE
914 South College
Tahlequah, OK 74464
(918) 456-0637
(800) 225-9868
Fax: (918) 453-0133

CHOCTAW
PO Box 638
1602 East Kirk
Hugo, OK 74743
(580) 326-3325
(800) 225-0076
Fax: (580) 326-3453

CIMARRON
PO Box 326
One Courthouse Square
Boise City, OK 73933
(580) 544-2512
(800) 572-6838
Fax: (580) 544-2707

CLEVELAND
631 East Robinson
Norman, OK 73071
(405) 321-1434
(800) 572-6823
Fax: (405) 364-1764

COAL
One North Main Street
Coalgate, OK 74538
(580) 927-2379
(800) 572-6829
Fax: (580) 927-2342

COMANCHE
2609 South West Lee Boulevard.
Lawton, OK 73505
(580) 250-3600
(800) 572-6841
Fax: (580) 250-3740

COTTON
1st Floor, Courthouse
Walters, OK 73572
(580) 875-6131
(800) 572-6830
Fax: (580) 875-3624

CRAIG
310 North Wilson
Vinita, OK 74301
(918) 256-8711
(800) 572-6844
Fax: (918) 256-8257

CREEK
17 South Elm
Sapulpa, OK 74066
(918) 224-0213
(800) 572-6834
Fax: (918) 224-0849

CUSTER
190 South 31st Street
Clinton, OK 73601
(580) 323-3333
(800) 572-6846
Fax: (580) 323-7204

DELAWARE
PO Drawer 750
Highway 59 South
Jay, OK 74346
(918) 253-4213
(800) 433-6772
Fax: (918) 253-6534

DEWEY
PO Box 128
Courthouse Basement
Taloga, OK 73667
(580) 328-5546
(800) 433-6967
Fax: (580) 328-5524

ELLIS
PO Box 215
103 North Washington
Arnett, OK 73832
(580) 885-7546
(800) 433-6773
Fax: (580) 885-7490

GARFIELD
PO Box 3628
2405 Mercer Drive
Enid, OK 73702
(580) 548-2100
(800) 433-7074
Fax: (580) 242-6535

GARVIN
Rt. 1, Box 34
Pauls Valley, OK 73075
(405) 238-6461
(800) 433-6846
Fax: (405) 238-9554

GRADY
217 North 3rd Street
Chickasha, OK 73018
(405) 224-2733
(800) 433-7075
Fax: (405) 222-0117

GRANT
112 East Guthrie
Room 303 / Courthouse
Medford, OK 73759
(580) 395-3312
(800) 433-6909
Fax: (580) 395-2815

GREER
130 North Oklahoma
Mangum, OK 73554
(580) 782-3311
(800) 433-7076
Fax: (580) 782-2051

HARMON
Courthouse, First Floor, Room 6
114 West Hollis
Hollis, OK 73550
(580) 688-3361
(800) 433-6945
Fax: (580) 688-2367

HASKELL
PO Box 659
#9 Highway East
Stigler, OK 74462
(918) 967-4658
(800) 638-3641
Fax: (918) 967-8647

HUGHES
801 Kingsberry
Holdenville, OK 74848
(405) 379-7231
(800) 493-7980
Fax: (405) 379-2376

JACKSON
1220 North Grady
Altus, OK 73521
(580) 482-5812
(800) 493-7974

JEFFERSON
212 South Main
Waurika, OK 73573
(580) 228-3581
(800) 493-7981
Fax: (580) 228-3626

JOHNSTON
Rt. 1, Box 94
1009 East Main, Suite 4
Tishomingo, OK 73460
(580) 371-2314
(800) 493-7975
Fax: (580) 371-2649

KAY
PO Box 210
801 West South Street
Newkirk, OK 74647
(580) 362-2548
(800) 597-1872
Fax: (580) 362-4179

KINGFISHER
PO Box 118
102 West Coronado
Kingfisher, OK 73750
(405) 375-3867
(800) 493-7976
Fax: (405) 375-6493

KIOWA
507 South Washington
Hobart, OK 73651
(580) 726-3339
(800) 493-7983
Fax: (580) 726-3622

LATIMER
PO Box 609
1809 Highway 270 East
Wilburton, OK 74578
(918) 465-2333
(800) 493-7978
Fax: (918) 465-3513

LE FLOR
PO Box 370
511 South Harper
Poteau, OK 74953
(918) 649-2300
(800) 493-7960
Fax: (918) 649-2481

LINCOLN
Courthouse
811 Manvel, Suite 1
Chandler, OK 74834
(405) 258-1680
(800) 493-7984
Fax: (405) 258-5231

LOGAN
219 South Broad
Guthrie, OK 73044
(405) 282-4500
(800) 572-6831
Fax: (405) 282-4555

LOVE
311 South Highway 77
Suite A
Marietta, OK 73448
(580) 276-3383
(800) 815-7558
Fax: (580) 276-5413

MAJOR
PO Box 98
1425 North Main, Suite 3,4,and 5
Fairview, OK 73737
(580) 227-3759
(800) 815-7571
Fax: (580) 227-2368

MARSHALL
403 East Main
Madill, OK 73446
(580) 795-7361
(800) 815-7567
Fax: (580) 795-5918

MAYES
501 South Elliott
Pryor, OK 74361
(918) 825-4535
(800) 815-7572
Fax: (918) 825-0441

MC CLAIN
PO Box 467
2148 South Green Avenue
Purcell, OK 73080
(405) 527-6511
(800) 815-7570
Fax: (405) 527-2085

MC CURTAIN
PO Box 329
1300 South East Adams
Idabel, OK 74745
(580)286-6581
(800) 815-7562
Fax: (580)286-6149

MCINTOSH
PO Box 231
Hospital Road & Highway 69
Eufaula, OK 74432
(918) 689-2524
(800) 219-3238
Fax: (918) 689-9786

MURRAY
1019 West Wyandotte
Sulphur, OK 73086
(580) 622-2186
(800) 815-7568
Fax: (580) 622-3734

MUSKOGEE
727 South 32nd
Muskogee, OK 74401
Mail to: PO Box 608
Muskogee, OK 74402
(918) 684-5300
(800) 815-7573
Fax: (918) 684-5377

NOBLE
205 15th Street
Perry, OK 73077
(580) 336-5581
(800) 815-7569
Fax: (580) 336-4795

NOWATA
309 Delaware
Nowata, OK 74048
(918) 273-2327
(800) 815-7574
Fax: (918) 273-1748

OKFUSKEE
119 South First
Okemah, OK 74859
(918) 623-1363
(800) 884-1528
Fax: (918) 623-9169

OKLAHOMA 55A
401 West Commerce
Oklahoma City, OK 73109
(405) 644-5700
(800) 884-1532
Fax: (405) 634-5824

OKLAHOMA 55B
7430 South East 15th
MidWest City, OK 73110
(405) 739-8000
(800) 884-1579
Fax: (405) 739-8132

OKLAHOMA 55C
PO Box 26768
2409 North Kelley Avenue
Oklahoma City, OK 73126
(405) 522-5818
(800) 884-1534
Fax: (405) 427-8548

OKLAHOMA 55D
5905 North Classen
Oklahoma City, OK 73118
(405) 713-6853
(800) 884-1581
Fax: (405) 713-6749

OKLAHOMA 55E
PO Box 26307
940 NE 13th (73104)
Oklahoma City, OK 73126
(405) 271-3325
(800) 884-1572
Fax: (405) 271-3338

OKMULGEE
5005 North Wood Drive
Okmulgee, OK 74447
(918) 752-2000
(800) 884-1582
Fax: (918) 752-2090

OSAGE
550 Kihekah
Pawhuska, OK 74056
(918) 287-2956
(800) 884-1573
Fax: (918) 287-1524

OTTAWA
1601 North Main
Miami, OK 74354
(918) 542-2836
(800) 884-1715
Fax: (918) 540-0913

PAWNEE
501 5th Street
Pawnee, OK 74058
(918) 762-3606
(800) 270-0786
Fax: (918) 762-3476

PAYNE
711 East Krayler
Stillwater, OK 74075
(405) 372-1941
(800) 270-0797
Fax: (405) 624-7304

PITTSBURG
PO Box 1006
1210 East Cherokee
McAlester, OK 74502
(918) 423-3066
(800) 270-0792
Fax: (918) 423-0174

PONTOTOC
1628 East Beverly, Suite 104
Ada, OK 74820
(580) 310-7050
(800) 270-0798
Fax: (580) 310-7051

POTTAWATOMIE
1400 North Kennedy
Shawnee, OK 74801
(405) 878-4000
(800) 270-0793

PUSHMATAHA
PO Box 40
104 South East "B" Street
Antlers, OK 74523
(580) 298-3361
(800) 270-0803
Fax: (580) 298-2129

ROGER MILLS
PO Box 339
480 East Broadway
Cheyenne, OK 73628
(580) 497-3393
(800) 270-0794
Fax: (580) 497-2632

SEMINOLE
206 East Second
Wewoka, OK 74884-2604
(405) 257-6651
(800) 270-0796
Fax: (405) 257-5135

Satellite Office:
111 North 4th Street
Seminole, OK 74868
(405) 382-6050
Fax: (405) 382-5977

SEQUOYAH
HC61, Box 20
Highway 59 (South of 1-40)
Sallisaw, OK 74955
(918) 775-4464
(800) 270-0805
Fax: (918) 775-5569

STEPHENS
PO Box 1367
1805 West Plato Road
Duncan, OK 73534
(580) 255-7550
(800) 734-7506
Fax: (580) 252-3621

TEXAS
1000 NE Fourth Street
Guymon, OK 73942
(580) 338-8592
(800) 734-7514
Fax: (580) 338-2988

TILLMAN
125 North Ninth
Frederick, OK 73542
580) 335-5537
(800) 734-7507
Fax: (580) 335-2856

TULSA (B)
3666 North Peoria
Tulsa, OK 74106
(918) 428-6304
(800) 734-7509
Fax: (918) 428-5613

TULSA (C)
444 South Houston
Tulsa, OK 74127
(918) 581-2401
(800) 734-7516
Fax: (918) 581-2500

Satellite Office:
320 East Midway
PO Box 2440
Broken Arrow, OK 74013
(918) 251-5251
Fax: (918) 251-5529

TULSA (G)
5051 South 129th East Avenue
Tulsa, OK 74134
(918) 294-2000

WAGONER
102 North East Seventh
Wagoner, OK 74467
(918) 485-4543
(800) 734-7518
Fax: (918) 485-5941

WASHINGTON
PO Box 1099 (74005)
700 South Penn
Bartlesville, OK 74003
(918) 336-2655
(800) 734-7512
Fax: (918) 336-6329

WASHITA
106 Lowber Lane
Cordell, OK 73632
(580) 832-3391
(800) 734-7519
Fax: (580) 832-3516

WOODS
1616 Oklahoma Boulevard
PO Box 724
Alva, OK 78717
(580) 327-2714
(800) 734-7513
Fax: (580) 327-4204

WOODS
4900 West Oklahoma
Woodward, OK 73801
(580) 256-6091
(800) 734-7520
Fax: (580) 254-5462

OREGON

ADULT AND FAMILY SERVICES DIVISION
500 Summer Street, NE-Salem, OR 97310-1013

DISTRICT 1 OFFICE
450 Marine Drive, Suite 200
PO Box 88
Astoria, OR 97103
(503) 325-2021

SAINT HELENS
500 North Highway 30, Suite 210
Street Helens, OR 97051
(503) 397-1784

ASTORIA
450 Marine Drive, Suite 200
PO Box 88
Astoria, OR 97103
(503) 325-2021

TILLAMOOK
3600 East 3rd Street
Tillamook, OR 97141
(503) 842-4453

DISTRICT 2 OFFICE
3965 South East Powell
Portland, OR 97202
(503) 731-3111

SOUTH EAST PORTLAND
3975 South East Powell
PO Box 86469
Portland, OR 97286
(503) 731-3181

ALBINA
30 North Webster
PO Box 11334
Portland, OR 97211
(503) 280-6781

BEAVERTON
12901 South West Jenkins Road, Suite B
PO Box 4007
Beaverton, OR 97005
(503) 646-9952

EAST PORTLAND
1415 South East 122nd
PO Box 16817
Portland, OR 97292
(503) 257-4200

GRESHAM
1415 South East 122nd
Portland, OR 97233
(503) 257-4449

HILLSBORO
1657 South East Enterprise Circle, Suite 100
PO Box 1687
Hillsboro, OR 97123
(503) 693-1833

NORTH EAST PORTLAND
4425 North East Broadway
PO Box 13790
Portland, OR 97213
(503) 280-6683

OUTER SOUTHEAST PORTLAND
1415 South East 122nd
Portland, OR 97233
(503) 257-4226

TIGARD
10577 South West Cascade Avenue
PO Box 231268
Beaverton, OR 97223
(503) 646-9952

WEST PORTLAND
10 North West 3rd
PO Box 3230
Portland, OR 97208
(503) 731-8383

CENTRAL OFFICE
500 Summer Street North East
Salem, OR 97310-1013
(503) 945-5600

DISTRICT 3 OFFICE
4074 Winema North East
Suite 101, Building 53
PO Box 17909
Salem, OR 97305
(503) 378-3402

NORTH SALEM
4074 Winema North East
Suite 101, Building 53
PO Box 17909
Salem, OR 97305
(503) 378-2731

DALLAS
177 South West Oak Street
PO Box 85
Dallas, OR 97338
(503) 623-5526

INDEPENDENCE
1605 Monmouth Street
Independence, OR 97351
(503) 838-0584

MCMINNVILLE
330 Kirby
PO Box 417
McMinnville, OR 97128
(503) 472-0311

SOUTH SALEM
1185 22nd Avenue South East
PO Box 14200
Salem, OR 97309
(503) 378-6327

SANTIAM CENTER
11656 Sublimity Road South East, Suite 200
PO Box 278
Stayton, OR 97385-9650
(503) 769-7439

WOODBURN
2200 Country Club Court
Woodburn, OR 97071
(503) 982-9991

DISTRICT 4 OFFICE
118 South East 2nd, Suite C
Albany, OR 97321
(541) 967-2179

ALBANY
118 South East 2nd, Suite C
Albany, OR 97321
(541) 967-2078

CORVALLIS
545 South West Second, #B
Corvallis, OR 97333
Ph. (541) 757-4201

LEBANON
320 Market Street
Lebanon, OR 97355
(541) 451-1050

NEWPORT
120 North East Avery Street
Newport, OR 97365
(541) 265-2248

DISTRICT 5
2885 Chad Drive
Eugene, OR 97408
(541) 687-7373

COTTAGE GROVE
260 Gateway Blvd
PO Box 876
Cottage Grove, OR 97424
(541) 942-9186

EUGENE
2885 Chad Drive
Eugene, OR 97408
(541) 686-7878

FLORENCE
3180 Highway 101
PO Box U
Florence, OR 97439
(541) 997-8251

JUNCTION CITY
225 West 6th
PO Box 22808
Junction City, OR 97402
(541) 997-8251

SPRINGFIELD
101 30th Street
Springfield, OR 97477
(541) 726-3525

WEST EUGENE
2175 West 7th
PO Box 22808
Eugene, OR 97402
(541) 686-7722

DISTRICT 6
1937 West Harvard Blvd
PO Box 70
Roseburg, OR 97470
(541) 440-3301

DRAIN FAMILY CENTER
129 West C Stree
PO Box 361
Drain, OR 97435
(541) 836-2939

ROSEBURG
1937 West Harvard Blvd
PO Box 70
Roseburg, OR 97470
(541) 440-3301

DISTRICT 7
2110 Newmark
Coos Bay, OR 97420
(541) 888-7045

COOS BAY
2110 Newmark
Coos Bay, OR 97420
(541) 888-7047

COOS AND CURRY COUNTIES ONE STOP
2110 Newmark
Coos Bay, OR 97420
(541) 888-2667

GOLD BEACH
94145 West 5th Place
PO Box 616
Gold Beach, OR 97444
(541) 247-7036

DISTRICT 8
800 Cardley Avenue
PO Box 1190
Medford, OR 97504
(541) 776-6186

ASHLAND
1658 Ashland Street
Ashland, OR 97520
(541) 482-2041

CAVE JUNCTION
228 North Redwood Highway
Cave Junction, OR 97523
(541) 592-4149

GRANTS PASS
726 North East 7th
Grants Pass, OR 97526
(541) 474-3101

MEDFORD
800 Cardley Avenue
PO Box 1190
Medford, OR 97501
(541) 776-6172

ROGUE FAMILY CENTER
2400 Antelope Rd
PO Box 2570
White City, OR 97503
(541) 830-8226

CHILD CARE NETWORK
673 Market Street
Medford, OR 97504
(541) 776-5100

DISTRICT 9
700 Union Street
The Dalles, OR 97058
(541) 296-4661

CONDON
425 North Washington
PO Box 65
Condon, OR 97823
(541) 384-2882

HOOD RIVER
910 Pacific Avenue, Suite 400
Hood River, OR 97031
(541) 386-3199

THE DALLES
700 Union Street
The Dalles, OR 97058
(541) 296-4661

DISTRICT 10
247 SouthEast Salmon, Suite A
Redmond, OR 97756
(541) 548-5547

BEND
1001 South West Emkay Drive, Suite A
Bend, OR 97702
(541) 388-6010

LAPINE
16493 Bluewood Place Units 3 and 4
PO Box 98
Lapine, OR 97739
(541) 536-5380

MADRAS
678 North East Highway 97, Suite A
Madras, OR 97741
(541) 475-6131

PRINEVILLE
1495 North East 3rd Street, Suite A
Prineville, OR 97754
(541) 447-3851

REDMOND
247 South East Salmon, Suite A
Redmond, OR 97756
(541) 548-5547

DISTRICT 11
700 Klamath Avenue, Suite 100
Klamath Falls, OR 97601
(541) 883-5542

KLAMATH FALLS
700 Klamath Avenue, Suite 100
Klamath Falls, OR 97601
(541) 883-5511

LAKEVIEW
108 E Street North, Suite 101
Lakeview, OR 97630
(541) 947-3376

DISTRICT 12
950 South East Columbia, Suite A
Hermiston, OR 97838
(541) 564-5673

HEPPNER
120 South Main
Heppner, OR 97836
(541) 676-5569

HERMISTON
950 South East Columbia, Suite A
Hermiston, OR 97838
(541) 564-5674

MILTON-FREEWATER
309 North Columbia
Milton-Freewater, OR 97862
(541) 938-6627

PENDLETON
700 South East Emigrant, Suite 120
Pendleton, OR 97801
(541) 276-9000

DISTRICT 13
1768 Auburn Street
Baker City, OR 97814
(541) 523-3648

BAKER CITY
1768 Auburn Street
Baker City, OR 97814
(541) 523-3648

ENTERPRISE
502 South River Street
PO Box A
Enterprise, OR 97828
(541) 426-3146

JOHN DAY
725 West Main Street, Suite A
John Day, OR 97845
(541) 575-0309

LAGRANDE
1901 Adams Avenue
LaGrande, OR 97850
(541) 963-4113

DISTRICT 14
702 Sunset Drive, Suite 100
Ontario, OR 97914
(541) 889-9141

BURNS
809 West Jackson, Suite 100
Burns, OR 97720
(541) 573-5227

ONTARIO
702 Sunset Drive, Suite 100
Ontario, OR 97914
(541) 889-9141

DISTRICT 15
315 South Beavercreek Road
PO Box 1520
Oregon City, OR 97045-8120
(503) 657-2151

OREGON CITY
315 South Beavercreek Road
PO Box 5120
Oregon City, OR 97045-8120
(503) 657-2152

MILWAUKIE
4252 South East Intl Way, Suite A
PO Box 22470
Milwaukie, OR 97269
(503) 731-4242

OREGON HEALTH PLAN
2850 Broadway NE
Salem, OR 97303
(800) 943-9249

DIRECT PAY UNIT
2850 Broadway NE
Keizer, OR 97303
(503) 373-0727 or (800) 442-6451

CLIENT MAINTENANCE
2850 Broadway NE
Keizer, OR 97303
(503) 378-4369

PENNSYLVANIA

ADAMS COUNTY
PO Box 4446
225 South Franklin Street
Gettysburg, PA 17325-4446
717-334-6241
1-800-638-6816
fax 717-334-4104

ALLEGHENY COUNTY
611 Pittsburgh State Office Building
300 Liberty Avenue
Pittsburgh, PA 15222-1215
142-565-2146
fax 412-565-3660

ALLE-KISKI DISTRICT
909 Industrial Blvd
New Kensington, PA 15068
724-339-6815
fax 724-339-6850

EASTERN DISTRICT
5919 Penn Avenue
Pittsburgh, PA 15206
412-645-6400
fax 412-645-7009

INSTITUTION RELATED ELIGIBILITY DISTRICT (IRED)
531 Penn Avenue
Pittsburgh, PA 15206
412-645-6400
fax 412-645-7009

LIBERTY DISTRICT
610 Wood Street
Pittsburgh, PA 15222-2513
412-565-2652
fax 412-565-5088

NORTH COUNTY
400 Stanwix Street
Room 800
Pittsburgh, PA 15222
412-565-7755 or 412-565-7756
fax 412-565-5198

NORTHERN DISTRICT
400 Stanwix Street
Room 600
Pittsburgh, PA 15222
412-565-5638
fax 412-565-5075

SOUTH SIDE DISTRICT
2100 Wharton Square
Pittsburgh, PA 15203
412-488-2030 or 412-488-7806
fax 412-488-6986

SOUTHEAST DISTRICT
220 Sixth Street
McKeesport, PA 15132-2720
412-664-6800 or 412-664-6801
fax 412-664-5218

SOUTHERN DISTRICT
300 Liberty Avenue
9th floor
Pittsburgh, PA 15222-1217
412-565-2232
fax 412-565-5179

SUSQUEHANNA DISTRICT
5947 Penn Avenue
Pittsburgh, PA 15206-3844
412-645-7400 or 412-645-7401
fax 412-645-7008

ARMSTRONG COUNTY
1280 North Water Street
Kittanning, PA 16201-0898
724-543-1651
1-800-424-5235
fax 724-548-0274

BEAVER COUNTY
171 Virginia Avenue
PO Box 349
Rochester, PA 15074-0349
724-773-7300
fax 724-773-7859

BEDFORD COUNTY
608 East Pitt Street
PO Box 163
Bedford, PA 15522-9975
814-624-4002
1-800-542-8584
fax 814-623-7310

BERKS COUNTY
Reading State Office Building
625 Cherry Street
Reading, PA 19602-1188
610-763-4211
fax 610-736-4004

BLAIR COUNTY
1100 Green Avenue
Altoona, PA 16601-3440
814-946-7111
1-800-532-0319
fax 814-941-6813

BRADFORD COUNTY
715 Main Street
PO Box 398
Towanda, PA 18848-0398
570-265-9186
1-800-542-3938
fax 570-265-3061

BUCKS COUNTY
1214 New Rodgers Road
Bristol, PA 19007-2593
215-781-3300
fax 215-781-3438

WARMINISTER DISTRICT
1386 West Street Road
Warminister, PA 18974-3111
215-443-3200
1-800-362-1291
fax 215-443-3208

BUTLER COUNTY
108 Woody Drive
PO Box 1590
Butler, PA 16003-1590
724-284-8844
fax 724-284-8833

CAMBRIA COUNTY
239 Main Street
Johnstown, PA 15901-1678
814-533-2491
fax 814-533-2214

CARBON COUNTY
80 Susquehanna Street
Jim Thorpe, PA 18229-0169
570-325-9540
fax 570-325-9543

CENTRE COUNTY
2580 Park Center Boulevard
State College, PA 16801-3005
814-863-6571
1-800-355-6024
fax 814-863-6585

CHESTER COUNTY
100 James Buchanan Drive
Thorndale, PA 19372
610-466-1000
1-800-814-4698
fax 610-466-1130

CLARION COUNTY
R. R. 3, Box 146B
PO Box 629
Clarion, PA 16214-0629
814-226-1700
1-800-253-3488
fax 814-226-1794

CLEARFIELD COUNTY
1121 Linden Street
Clearfield, PA 16830-3395
814-765-7591
1-800-521-9218
fax 814-765-0802

CLINTON COUNTY
220 Woodward Avenue
PO Box 450
Lock Haven, PA 17745-9987
570-748-2971
1-800-820-4159
fax 570-893-2973

COLUMBIA COUNTY
27 East Seventh Street
PO Box 628
Bloomsburg, PA 17815-0628
570-387-4200
1-877-211-1322
fax 570-387-4708

CRAWFORD COUNTY
1084 Water Street
PO Box 1187
Meadville, PA 16335-7187
814-333-3400
1-800-527-7861
fax 814-333-3527

CUMBERLAND COUNTY
33 Westminster Drive
PO Box 599
Carlisle, PA 17013-0599
717-240-2700
1-800-269-0173
fax 717-249-0919

DAUPHIN COUNTY
2432 North 7th Street
PO Box 5959
Harrisburg, PA 17110-0959
717-787-2324
1-800-788-5616
fax 717-772-4703

DELAWARE COUNTY
701 Crosby Street
Suite A
Chester, PA 19013-6099
610-447-5500
fax 610-447-5399

CROSBY DISTRICT
701 Crosby Street
Suite A
Chester, PA 19013-6099
610-447-5300

LANSDOWNE DISTRICT
77 South Union Avenue
Lansdowne, PA 19050-3026
610-284-6900
fax 610-284-7532

ELK COUNTY
301 North Broad Street
PO Box F
Ridgway, PA 15853-0327
814-776-1101
1-800-847-0257
fax 814-772-7007

ERIE COUNTY
1316 Holland Street
PO Box 958
Erie, PA 16512-0958
814-461-2000
1-800-635-1014
fax 814-461-2294

FAYETTE COUNTY
41 West Church Street
Uniontown, PA 15401-3418
724-439-7015
1-877-832-7545
fax 724-439-7002

FOREST COUNTY
Tionesta Towne House-Rear
Elm Street
PO Box 367
Tionesta, PA 16353-0367
814-755-3552
1-800-876-0645
fax 814-755-3420

FRANKLIN COUNTY
620 Norland Avenue
Chambersburg, PA 17201-3496
717-264-6121
1-800-921-8839
fax 717-264-4801

FULTON COUNTY
Penn Village Shopping Plaza
Route 16
PO Box 637
McConnellsburg, PA 17233-0637
717-485-3151
1-800-222-8563
fax 717-485-3713

GREENE COUNTY
35 South West Street
PO Box 950
Waynesburg, PA 15370-0950
724-627-8171
1-888-410-5658
fax 724-627-8096

HUNTINGDON COUNTY
101 South Fifth Street
PO Box 398
Huntingdon, PA 16652-0398
814-643-1170
1-800-237-7674
fax 814-643-5441

INDIANA COUNTY
2750 Route 422 West
PO Box 728
Indiana, PA 15701-0728
724-357-2900
1-800-742-0679
fax 724-357-2951

JEFFERSON COUNTY
100 Prushnok Drive
PO Box 720
Punxsutawney, PA 15767
814-93802990
1-800-242-8214
fax 814-938-3842

JUNIATA COUNTY
100 Meadow Lane
PO Box 65
Mifflintown, PA 17059-9983
717-436-2158
1-800-586-4282
fax 717-436-5402

LACKAWANNA COUNTY
200 Scranton State Office Building
100 Lackawanna Avenue
Scranton, PA 18503-1972
570-963-4525
1-877-431-1887
fax 570-963-4843

LANCASTER COUNTY
832 Manor Street
PO Box 4967
Lancaster, PA 17604-4967
717-299-7411
fax 717-299-7565

LAWRENCE COUNTY
108 East South Street
New Castle, PA 16101-3888
724-656-3000
1-800-847-4522
fax 724-656-3076

LEBANON COUNTY
625 South 8th Street
PO Box 870
Lebanon, PA 17042-0870
717-270-6721
1-800-229-3926
fax 717-228-2589

LEHIGH COUNTY
101 South 7th
Allentown, PA 18101-2295
610-821-6509
fax 610-821-6705

LUZERNE COUNTY
85 East Union Street
Wilkes-Barre, PA 18711-3298
570-826-2100
fax 570-820-4876

WILKES-BARRE DISTRICT
85 East Union Street
Wilkes-Barre, PA 18711-3298
570-826-2100

HAZLETON DISTRICT
Center Plaza Building
10 West Chestnut Street
Hazleton, PA 18201-6409
570-459-3800
fax 570-459-3931

LYCOMING COUNTY
400 Little League Boulevard
PO Box 127
Williamsport, PA 17703-0127
570-327-3300
1-877-867-4014
fax 570-321-6501

MCKEAN COUNTY
90 Boylston Street
PO Box 16
Bradford, PA 16701-0016
814-362-4671
1-800-822-1108
814-362-4959

MERCER COUNTY
2236 Highland Road
Hermitage, PA 16148-2896
724-983-5000
1-800-747-8405
fax 724-983-5706

MIFFLIN COUNTY
1125 Riverside Drive
PO Box 1942
Lewistown, PA 17044-1942
717-248-6746
1-800-382-5253
fax 717-242-6099

MONROE COUNTY
Business Route 209 South at
Tanite Road
PO Box 232
Stroudsburg, PA 18360-0232
570-424-3030
fax 570-424-3915

MONTGOMERY/NORRISTOWN DISTRICT
1950 Calamia Drive
Norristown, PA 19401-3191
610-270-3500
fax 610-270-1678

POTTSTOWN DISTRICT
19 North Charlotte Street
Pottstown, PA 19464-5584
610-327-4280
fax 610-327-4350

MONTOUR COUNTY
327 Church Street
PO Box 278
Danville, PA 17821-0278
570-275-7430
fax 570-275-7433

NORTHAMPTON COUNTY
201 Larry Holmes Drive
PO Box 10
Easton, PA 18044-0010
610-250-1700
fax 610-250-1839

NORTHUMBERLAND COUNTY
320 Chestnut Street
Sunbury, PA 17801
570-988-5900
1-800-368-8390
fax 570-988-5918

PERRY COUNTY
Cold Storage Road
PO Box 280
New Bloomfield, PA 17068-0280
717-582-2127
1-800-991-1929
fax 717-582-4187

PHILADELPHIA COUNTY
Philadelphia State Office Building
1400 Spring Garden Street
Philadelphia, PA 19130-4088
215-560-2900
fax 215-560-2114

ALDEN DISTRICT
5853 Germantown Avenue
Philadelphia, PA 19144-2154
215-560-4800
fax 215-560-4876

BOULEVARD DISTRICT
109 Frankford Avenue
Philadelphia, PA 19124-4508
215-560-6500
fax 215-560-2087

CENTER DISTRICT
900 N. Marshall Street
Philadelphia, PA 19123-1307
215-560-3600
fax 215-560-3648

DELANCEY DISTRICT
5548 Chestnut Street
1st floor
Philadelphia, PA 19139-3204
215-560-3700
fax 215-560-2055

ELMWOOD DISTRICT
5554 Chestnut Street
2nd floor
Philadelphia, PA 19139-3204
215-560-3800
fax 215-560-2065

FEDERAL DISTRICT
1415 Catherine Street
Philadelphia, PA 19146-2299
215-560-4400
fax 215-560-2066

GIRARD DISTRICT
961 North Marshall Street
Philadelphia, PA 19123-1306
215-560-3500
fax 215-560-6996

HILL DISTRICT
301 East Chelten Avenue
3rd floor
Philadelphia, PA 19144-5751
215-560-5200

JEFFERSON DISTRICT
2701 North Broad Street
3rd floor
Philadelphia, PA 19132-2743
215-560-6600
fax 215-560-2039

KENT DISTRICT
2701 North Broad Street
2nd floor
Philadelphia, PA 19132-2743
215-560-7100
fax 215-560-5403

LEHIGH DISTRICT
2701 North Broad Street
4th floor
Philadelphia, PA 19132-2743
215-560-4600
fax 215-560-2248

NORTH DISTRICT
219 East Lehigh Avenue
Philadelphia, PA 19125-1099
215-560-4000
fax 215-560-4065

NURSING HOME DISTRICT
4601 Market Street
Ground Floor
Philadelphia, PA 19139-4616
215-560-5500
fax 215-560-3469

OGONTZ DISTRICT
301 East Chelten Avenue
2nd floor
Philadelphia, PA 19144-5751
215-560-5000
fax 215-560-5116

RIDGE DISTRICT
1350 West Sedgley Avenue
Philadelphia, PA 19132-2496
215-560-4900
fax 215-560-4938

SNYDER DISTRICT
990 Buttonwood Street
5th floor
Philadelphia, PA 19123
215-560-4300
fax 215-560-4321

TIOGA DISTRICT
1348 West Sedgley Street
Philadelphia, PA 19132-2498
215-560-4700
fax 215-560-2260

UNITY DISTRICT
4111 Frankford Avenue
Philadelphia, PA 19124-4508
215-560-6400
fax 215-560-2067

VINE DISTRICT
4601 Market Street
1st floor
Philadelphia, PA 19139-4616
215-560-2301
fax 215-560-7818

WEST DISTRICT
5070 Parkside Avenue
Philadelphia, PA 19131-4747
215-560-6100
fax 215-560-2053

PIKE COUNTY
Suite 101
County Commerce Center
10 Buist Road
Milford, PA 18337-0027
570-296-6114
fax 570-296-4183

POTTER COUNTY
343 Port Allegany Road
Coudersport, PA 16915-9501
814-274-9700
1-800-446-9896
fax 814-274-8958

SCHUYLKILL COUNTY
2640 Woodglen Road
Pottsville, PA 17901-1341
570-621-3000
1-877-306-5439
fax 570-621-3014

SNYDER COUNTY
570 South High Street
PO Box 56
Selinsgrove, PA 17870-0056
570-374-8126
fax 570-374-6347

SOMERSET COUNTY
600 Aberdeen Drive
Somerset, PA 15501-1799
814-443-3681
1-800-248-1607
fax 814-445-4352

SULLIVAN COUNTY
268 Overton Road
PO Box 577
Dushore, PA 18624-0577
570-928-8596
1-877-265-1681
fax 570-928-8013

SUSQUEHANNA COUNTY
33 Spruce Street
PO Box 128
Montrose, PA 18801-0128
570-278-3891
1-888-753-6328
fax 570-278-9508

TIOGA COUNTY
144 E. East Avenue
Wellsboro, PA 16901-1738
570-724-4051
1-800-525-6842
fax 570-724-4927

UNION COUNTY
1610 Industrial Boulevard
Suite 300
Lewisburg, PA 17837-1273
570-524-2201
fax 570-524-2361

VENANGO COUNTY
1272 Elk Street
PO Box 391
Franklin, PA 16323-0391
814-437-4241 or 814-437-4242
1-800-522-2078
fax 814-437-4441

WARREN COUNTY
PO Box 397
Warren, PA 16365-0397
814-723-6330
1-800-403-4043
fax 1-814-726-1565

WASHINGTON COUNTY
167 North Main Street
PO Box 5004
Washington, PA 15301-1154
724-223-4300
1-800-835-9720
fax 724-223-4675

VALLEY DISTRICT
595 Galiffa Drive
PO Box 592
Donora, PA 15033-0592
724-379-1500
1-800-392-6932
fax 724-379-1572

WAYNE COUNTY
107 8th Street, 2nd floor
PO Box 229
Honesdale, PA 18431-0229
570-253-7111
1-877-879-5267
fax 570-253-7374

WESTMORELAND COUNTY
587 Sells Lane
Greensburg, PA 15601-4493
724-832-5200
1-800-905-5413
fax 724-832-5202

DONORA DISTRICT
595 Galiffa Drive
PO Box 592
Donora, PA 15033-0592
1-800-238-9094
fax 724-379-1572

ALLE-KISKI DISTRICT
909 Industrial Boulevard
New Kensington, PA 15068
1-800-622-3527
fax 724-339-6850

EAST GREENSBURG DISTRICT
595 Sells Lane
Greensburg, PA 15601
1-800-905-5413
fax 724-832-5329

WYOMING COUNTY
PO Box 490, Route 6
Tunkhannock, PA 18657-0490
570-836-5171
fax 570-836-8761

YORK COUNTY
130 North Duke Street
PO Box 15041
York, PA 17405-7041
717-771-1100
fax 717-771-1261

PUERTO RICO
We experienced difficulty in obtaining information. Please contact the following for details concerning Medicaid eligibility guidelines in Puerto Rico.

Puerto Rico Department of Health
PO Box 70184
San Juan, PR 00936-8184
(787) 274-7602
Public information officer (787) 274-7645
Fax: (787) 250-6547

Puerto Rico Office of Economic Aid to Medically Indigent/Medical Assistance Program

70 Ponce de Leon Avenue
Hato Rey, PR 00919
(787) 250-7429
Fax: (787) 250-0990

RHODE ISLAND
DEPARTMENT OF HUMAN SERVICES DISTRICT OFFICES

COVENTRY
65 Sandy Bottom Road
Coventry, RI 02816
(401) 828-2440

CRANSTON
600 New London Avenue
(401) 462-6500
Cranston & West Warwick Residents

EAST PROVIDENCE
75 James Street
East Providence, RI 02914
(401) 438-7500
East Providence, Barrington, Warren & Bristol residents

JOHNSTON
1514 Atwood Avenue
Johnston, RI 02919
(401) 222-5666
Johnston, Foster, North Providence, & Scituate residents

NEWPORT
12 Elm Street
Newport, RI 02840
(401) 849-6000
(800) 675-9397
Serving Newport, Portsmouth, Tiverton, Little Compton, Jamestown
& Middletown residents

NORTH KINGSTOWN
7734 Post Road
North Kingstown, RI 02852
(401) 884-7250
(800) 862-0222
North Kingstown, South Kingstown, & East Greenwich residents

PAWTUCKET
24 Commerce Street
Pawtucket, RI 02860
(401) 728-2000
(800) 984-8989
Pawtucket & Central Falls residents

PROVIDENCE
206 Elmwood Avenue
Providence, RI
(401) 222-7000

WARWICK
100 Meadow Street
Warwick, RI 02886
(401) 739-9530 and (401) 739-9540
(800) 471-1757

WESTERLY
10 Canal Street
Westerly, RI 02891
(401) 596-2081

WOONSOCKET
144 Main Street
Woonsocket, RI 02895
(401) 769-3500
Woonsocket, Cumberland, Lincoln, Smithfield, North Smithfield, Burrillville & Glocester residents

SOUTH CAROLINA COUNTY DEPARTMENTS OF SOCIAL SERVICES

ABBEVILLE
1 Human Services Bldg
903 West Greenwood Street
Abbeville, SC 29620
(864) 459-548

AIKEN
County Commissioner's Building
1410 Park Avenue South East
Post Office Drawer 1268
Aiken, SC 29802-1268
(803) 649-1111

ALLENDALE
103 Brandt Bldg
Courthouse Square
Allendale, SC 29810
(803) 584-7048

ANDERSON
Old Woolworth's Bldg
111 South Main Street
Post Office Box 827
Anderson, SC 29622-0827
(864) 260-4100

BAMBERG
Human Resources Center
#1 Log Branch Road
Post Office Box60
Bamberg, SC 29003
(803) 245-4363

BARNWELL
10913 Ellenton Street
Post Office Box 1306
Barnwell, SC 29812
(803) 541-1205

BEAUFORT
1905 Duke Street
Post Office Box 1065
Beaufort, SC 29901-1065
(843) 470-4569

BERKELEY
92 Belt Drive
Moncks Corner, SC 29461-2895
(843) 761-2779

CALHOUN
304 S.F.R. Huff Drive
Post Office Box 467
Street Matthews, SC 29135
(803) 874-3384

CHARLESTON
3366 Rivers Avenue
North Charleston, SC 29405-5714
792-0444

CHEROKEE
1434 North Limestone
Post Office Box 1369
Gaffney, SC 29342-1369
(864) 487-2704

CHESTER
Reedy Street
Post Office Box 488
Chester, SC 29706
(803) 377-8131

CHESTERFIELD
202 West Main Street
Post Office Box 269
Chesterfield, SC 29709
(843) 623-2147

CLARENDON
3 South Church Street
Manning, SC 29102
(803) 435-4305

COLLETON
219 South Lemacks Street
Post Office Box 440
Walterboro, SC 29488
(843) 549-6090

DARLINGTON
130 East Camden Avenue
Post Office Drawer 1377
Hartsville, SC 29551
(843) 398-4420

DILLON
Highway 34 West
Post Office Box 1307
Dillon, SC 29536
(843) 774-8284

DORCHESTER
903 Dukes Street
Post Office Box 906
Street George, SC 29477
(843) 563-4337

EDGEFIELD
500 West A. Reel Drive
Post Office Box 644
Edgefield, SC 29824
(803) 637-4040

FAIRFIELD
Highway 321 By Pass & Kinard Bridge Road
Post Office Box 210
Winnsboro, SC 29180
(803) 635-5502

FLORENCE
2685 South Irby Street
Box A
Florence, SC 29505
843) 669-3354

GEORGETOWN
330 Dozier Street
Georgetown, SC 29440
(843) 546-5134

GREENVILLE
County Square
301 University Ridge, Suite 6700
Post Office Box 10887
Greenville, SC 29603
(864) 467-7982

GREENWOOD
1118 Phoenix Street
Post Office Box 1096
Greenwood, SC 29648
(864) 229-5258

HAMPTON
T. Deloach Building
Room 126
201 Jackson Street
W Hampton, SC 29924
(803) 943-3641

HORRY
1951 Industrial Park Road
Conway, SC 29526
(843)365-5565

JASPER
Jacob Smart Boulevard
Corner of Highway 17 & Wilson Street
Post Office Box 1359
Ridgeland, SC 29936
726-7747

KERSHAW
County Social Services Bldg
816 DeKalb Street
Camden, SC 29020
(803) 432-7676

LANCASTER
1837 Pageland Highway
Human Services Complex
Post Office Box 1719
Lancaster, SC 29721
(803) 286-6914

LAURENS
Human Services Complex
Industrial Park Road
Post Office Box 2001
Laurens, SC 29360-2001
(864) 833-0100

LEE COUNTY
County Welfare Building
820 Brown Street
Post Office Box 389
Bishopville, SC 29010
(803) 484-6403

LEXINGTON
Social Services Center
541 Gibson Road
Post Office Drawer 430
Lexington SC 29071
957-7333

MCCORMICK
215 North Mine Street
Highway 28
North McCormick, SC 29835
(864) 465-2627

MARION
Beeson Building
180 Airport Road, Suite A
Post Office Box 1135
Mullins, SC 29574
(843)423-4623

MARLBORO
County Complex Ag Street
Post Office Drawer 120
Bennettsville, SC 29512
(843)479-4389

NEWBERRY
County Human Services Center
1306 Hunt Street
Post Office Box 309
Newberry, SC 29108
(803) 321-2155

OCONEE
100 Brown Square Drive
Post Office Box 739
Walhalla, SC 29691
(864)638-4400

ORANGEBURG
2570 Old Street Matthews Rd, NE
Post Office Box 1087
Orangeburg, SC 29116-1087
(803)531-3101

PICKENS
Social Services Building
McDaniel Avenue
Post Office Box 158
Pickens, SC 29671
(864)898-5810

RICHLAND
3220 Two Notch Road
Columbia, SC 29204
735-7048

SALUDA
Highway #121
North Post Office Box 276 3220
Saluda, SC 29138
(843) 445-2139

SPARTANBURG
Evans Human Resources Center |
142 South Dean
Post Office Drawer 3548
Spartanburg, SC 29304
(864)596-2292

SUMTER
105 North Magnolia Street
4th Floor, Post Office Box 68
Sumter, SC 29151-0068
(803) 773-5531

UNION
South Duncan By-pass
Post Office Box 428
Union, SC 29379
(843)429-1660

WILLIAMSBURG
1401 Eastland Avenue
Post Office Drawer 389
Kingstree, SC 29556
(843) 354-5411

YORK
Liberty Street
Post Office Box 261
York, SC 29745
(803) 684-8108

SOUTH DAKOTA
DEPARTMENT OF SOCIAL SERVICES FIELD OFFICES

I. CENTRAL DISTRICT

CHAMBERLAIN
PO Box 430
Chamberlain, SD 57325
(607) 734-6581
Fax: (607) 734-6284
Counties: Brule, Buffalo, Lyman

MISSION
PO Box 818
Mission, SD 57555-0818
(605) 856-4489
Fax: (605) 856-2031
Counties: Jones, Mellette, Todd

MOBRIDGE

PO Box 160
Mobridge, SD 57601-0160
(605) 845-2922
Fax: (605) 845-7126
Counties: Campbell, Corson, Dewey, Perkins, Potter, Walworth, Ziebach

PIERRE

912 East Sioux
C/O 500 East Capitol Avenue
Pierre, SD 57501-5070
(605) 773-3521
Fax: (605) 773-5390
Counties: Haakon, Hughes, Hyde, Stanley, Sully

WINNER

649 West Second Street
Winner, SD 575880-1598
(605) 842-0400
Fax: (605) 842-2574
Counties: Gregory, Tripp

II. NORHEASTERN DISTRICT

ABERDEEN

PO Box 1300
Aberdeen, SD 57402-1300
(605) 626-2381
Fax: (605) 626-2610
Counties: Brown, Edmunds, McPherson

BROOKINGS
PO Box 1408
Huron, SD 57350-1408
(605) 353-7105
Fax: (605) 353-7103
Counties: Beadle, Faulk, Hand

REDFIELD
Courthouse
210 East Seventh Avenue
Redfield, SD 57469-1299
(605) 472-4220
Fax: (605) 472-4298
Counties: Spink

SISSETON
PO Box 230
Sisseton, SD 572262-0230
(605) 698-7673
Fax: (605) 698-7842
Counties: Marshall, Roberts

WATERTOWN
PO Box 670
Watertown, SD 57201-0670
(605) 882-5000
Fax: (605) 886-6671
Counties: Clark, Codington, Deuel, Grant, Hamlin

WEBSTER
Courthouse
710 West First Street
Webster, SD 57274-1359
(605) 345-3432
Fax: (605) 345-4525
Counties: Day

III. SOUTHEASTERN DISTRICT

MITCHELL
PO Box 310
Mitchell, SD 57301-0310
(605) 995-8000
Fax: (605) 996-0681
Counties: Aurora, Charles Mix, Davison, Douglas, Hansen, Jerauld,
        Sanborn

SIOUX FALLS
300 East Sixth Street
Sioux Falls, SD 57103-7020
(605) 367-5600
Fax: (605) 367-5618
Counties: Lincoln, McCook, Minnehaha, Turner

VERMILLION
12 Court Street
Vermillion, SD 57069-0516
(605) 677-6800
Fax: (605) 677-6808
Counties: Clay, Union

YANKTON
3113 Spruce Street, Suite 200
Yankton, SD 57078-2726
(605) 668-3030
Fax: (605) 668-3014
Counties: Bon Homme, Hutchinson, Yankton

IV. WESTERN DISTRICT

DEADWOOD
PO Box 607
Deadwood, SD 57732-0607
(605) 578-2402
Fax: (605) 578-1280
Counties: Butte, Harding, Lawrence, Meade

HOT SPRINGS
2500 Minnekahta Avenue, Building 1
Hot Springs, SD 57747-0729
(605) 745-5100
Fax: (605) 745-6562
Counties: Custer, Fall River

PINE RIDGE
PO Box 279
Pine Ridge, SD 57770-0279
(605) 867-5861
Fax: (608) 867-2237
Counties: Bennett, Jackson, Shannon, Washabaugh

RAPID CITY
PO Box 2440
Rapid City, SD 57709-2440
(605) 394-2224
Fax: (605) 394-2568
Counties: Pennington

TENNESSEE DEPARTMENT OF HUMAN SERVICES DISTRICT/COUNTY OFFICES

ANDERSON COUNTY
District 1, Cty #1
PO Box 357 (37717-0357)
439 South Charles G.Seivers Blvd
Clinton, TN 37716-3511
(423) 457-3660
Fax: (423) 457-0335

BEDFORD COUNTY
District 5, Cty #2
PO Box 928
511 Madison Street
Shelbyville, TN 37160-3340
(931) 685-5006
Fax: (931) 685-5028

BENTON COUNTY
District 7, Cty #3
PO Box 897 (38320-0897)
216 North 641 Highway (38320-1330)
Camden, TN
(901) 584-4712
Fax: (901) 584-3055

BLEDSOE COUNTY
District 3, Cty #4
PO Box 396 (37367-0396)
218B North Main (37367)
Pikeville, TN
(423) 447-2193
Fax: (423) 447-6968

BLOUNT COUNTY
District 1, Cty #5
303 Home Avenue
Maryville, TN 37801-3920
(423) 981-2350
Fax: (423) 981-5685

BRADLEY COUNTY
District 3, Cty #6
950 Star Vue Drive, SW, Suite 1
Cleveland, TN 37311
(423) 478-0300
Fax: (423) 559-4986

CAMPBELL COUNTY
District 1, Cty #7
2247 Jacksboro Pike (37766-3003)
LaFollette, TN
(423) 566-9639
Fax: (423) 566-9734

CAMPBELL COUNTY BRANCH OFFICE
239 Broad Street
Jellico, TN 37762
(423) 784-9448
Fax: (423) 784-0995

CANNON COUNTY
District 3, Cty #8
PO Box 370 (37190-0370)
325 Bryant Lane
Woodbury, TN 37190-1629
(615) 563-4051
Fax: (615) 563-6262

CARROLL COUNTY
District 7, Cty #9
PO Box 526 (38344-0526)
20810 Main Street, East (38344-4203)
Huntingdon, TN
(901) 986-2211
Fax: (901) 986-8652

CARTER COUNTY
District 1, Cty #10
714 West C Street
Elizabethton, TN 37643-2590
(423) 543-3189
Fax: (423) 543-6559

CHEATHAM COUNTY
District 5, Cty #11
PO Box 218 (37015-0218)
1094 North Main Street (37015-1391)
Ashland City, TN
(615) 792-5628
Fax: (615) 792-9280

CHESTER COUNTY
District 7, Cty #12
1306 Highway 45
North Henderson, TN 38340-4003
(901) 989-5144
Fax: (901) 989-0422

CLAIBORNE COUNTY
District 1, Cty #13
PO Box 259 (37879-0259)
310 Court Street (37879-2001)
Tazewell, TN
(423) 626-7285
Fax: (423) 626-5092

CLAIBORNE COUNTY BRANCH OFFICE
PO Box 2 (37715-0002)
Highway 90, Box 1 (37715)
Clairfield, TN
(615) 784-4101

CLAY COUNTY
District 3, Cty #14
PO Box 448 (38551-0448)
141 East Lake Avenue (38551-4184)
Celina, TN
(931) 243-3183
Fax: (931) 243-4887

COCKE COUNTY
District 1, Cty #15
PO Box 1228 (37821-1228)
330 Heritage Blvd., Suite A (37821-4242)
Newport, TN
(423) 623-1291
Fax: (423) 625-4548

COFFEE COUNTY
District 5, Cty #16
PO Box 929 (37349-0929)
55 Saint Bede's Drive (37355)
Manchester, TN
(931) 723-5050
Fax: (931) 723-5061

CROCKETT COUNTY
District 7, Cty #17
PO Box 128 (38001-0128)
169 Cherry Street, North (38001-1102)
Alamo, TN
(901) 696-5441
Fax: (901) 696-3024

CUMBERLAND COUNTY
District 3, Cty #18
139 Cumberland Plaza
Crossville, TN 38555
(931) 484-2573
Fax: (931) 456-2961

DAVIDSON COUNTY
District 6, Cty #19
PO Box 1135 (37202-1135)
1000 2nd Avenue, North (37201-1028)
Nashville, TN
(615) 532-4000
Fax: (615) 741-7901 (Family Assistance)

MARTHA O'BRYAN RESOURCE CTR
711 South 7th Street
Nashville, TN 37206
(615) 862-6484

DISTRICT 5 NASHVILLE OFFICE
1616 Church Street Nashville, TN 37203-2920
(615) 741-3701
Fax: (615) 327-2241

STATE OFFICE
400 Deaderick Street
Nashville, TN 37248
(615) 313-4700
Fax: (615) 741-4165

DECATUR COUNTY
District 7, Cty #20
PO Box 8 (38329-0008)
42500 Highland Road(38329-9581)
Decaturville, TN
(901) 852-2981
Fax: (901) 852-4612

DEKALB COUNTY
District 7, Cty #21
1020 Broad Street,
West Smithville, TN 37166-2501
(615) 597-4725
Fax: (615) 597-8531

DICKSON COUNTY
District 5, Cty #22
222 State Street
Dickson, TN 37055-2084
(615) 441-6200
Fax: (615) 441-6185

DYER COUNTY
District 7, Cty #23
640 Highway 51 By-Pass East
Dyersburg, TN 38024-2067
(901) 286-8305
Fax: (901) 288-8008

FAYETTE COUNTY
District 7, Cty #24
PO Box 278 (38068-0278)
108 Kay Drive (38068-1210)
Somerville, TN
Phone: (901) 465-7334
Fax: (901) 465-7376

FENTRESS COUNTY
District 3, Cty #25
PO Box 68 (38556-0068)
342 Central Avenue, West (38556)
Jamestown, TN
(931) 879-9976
Fax: (931) 879-2955

FRANKLIN COUNTY
District 5, Cty #26
PO Box 560 (37398-0560)
708 South College Street (37398-2212)
Winchester, TN
(931) 962-1150
Fax: (931) 962-1141

GIBSON COUNTY
District 7, Cty #27
PO Box 188 (38382-0188)
1246A Manufacturer's Row (38382-3637)
Trenton, TN
(901) 855-7800
Fax: (901) 855-7855

DISTRICT 7 TRENTON OFFICE
1263 Highway 45 Bypass, North
Trenton, TN 38382-4006
(901) 855-7809
Fax: (901) 855-7854

GILES COUNTY
District 5, Cty #28
PO Box 902 (38478-0902)
219 Village Square (38478-2929)
Pulaski, TN
(931) 424-4001
Fax: (931) 424-4031

GRAINGER COUNTY
District 1, Cty #29
PO Box 188 (37861-0188)
Finley Bldg., 2188 Highway 11, West (37861)
Rutledge, TN
(423) 828-5245
Fax: (423) 828-4114

GREENE COUNTY
District 1, County #30
PO Box 189 (37744-0189)
128 Serral Drive (37744)
Greeneville, TN
(423) 639-6181
Fax: (423) 787-1496

GRUNDY COUNTY
District 3, Cty #31
PO Box 399 (37387-0399)
Highway 41 North, 606 Orchard Road 37387
Tracy City, TN
Phone: (931) 592-9231
Fax: (931) 592-9250

HAMBLEN COUNTY
District 1, Cty #32
2416 West Andrew Johnson Highway
Morristown, TN 37814
(423) 585-1444
Fax: (423) 587-7048

HAMILTON COUNTY
District 4, Cty #33
311 East Martin Luther King Blvd.
Chattanooga, TN 37403
(423) 634-6200
Fax: (423) 634-5868 or Fax: (423) 634-3141

DISTRICT OFFICE
311 East Martin Luther King Blvd
Chattanooga, TN 37403-4108
(423) 634-6355
Fax: (423) 634-6760

BRANCH OFFICE
540 McCallie Avenue
Chattanooga, TN 37402
Fax: (423) 634-6183

HAMILTON COUNTY
Main Street Issuance
2210 Main Street, East
Chattanooga, TN 37404-5296
(423) 634-3107

HAMILTON COUNTY
Alton Park Issuance
100 East 37th Street
Chattanooga, TN 37410-1498
(423) 634-3088

HANCOCK COUNTY
District 1, Cty #34
PO Box 6 (37869-0006)
210 West Main Street (37869)
Sneedville, TN
(423) 733-2401
Fax: (423) 733-1468

HARDEMAN COUNTY
District 7, Cty #35
PO Box 247 (38008-0247)
795 Tennessee Street
Bolivar, TN (38008)
(901) 658-5545
Fax: (901) 658-1559

HARDIN COUNTY
District 7, Cty #36
2100 Wayne Road
Savannah, TN 38372-2238
(901) 925-4968
Fax: (901) 926-1620

HAWKINS COUNTY
District 1, Cty #37
PO Box 910 (37857-0910)
4071 Highway 66, Suite 14 (37857)
Rogersville, TN
(423) 272-2606
Fax: (423) 272-5349

HAYWOOD COUNTY
District 7, Cty #38
1199 South Dupree
Brownsville, TN 38012-3235
(901) 772-4242
Fax: (901) 779-0151

HENDERSON COUNTY
District 7, Cty #39
PO Box 70 (38351-0070)
337 Church Street, West (38351-2017)
Lexington, TN
(901) 968-3652
Fax: (901) 968-6164

HENRY COUNTY
District 7, Cty #40
PO Box 430 (38242-0430)
1303 Wood Street, West (38242-5717)
Paris, TN
(901) 644-7350
Fax: (901) 644-7400

HENRY COUNTY REHAB SERVICE SOUTH OFFICE
508 North Market
Paris, TN 38242
(901) 644-7361

HICKMAN COUNTY
District 5, Cty #41
108 Progress Center Plaza
Centerville, TN 37033-1048
(931) 729-4212
Fax: (931) 729-9968

HOUSTON COUNTY
District 5, Cty #42
PO Box 269 (37061-0269)
501 Roby Drive (37061-9447)
Erin, TN
Phone: (931) 289-4105
Fax: (931) 289-4104

HUMPHREYS COUNTY
District 5, Cty #43
1203 Highway 70 West (37185-1437)
Waverly, TN
(931) 296-4227
Fax: (931) 296-2791

JACKSON COUNTY
District 3, Cty #44
PO Box 295 (38562-0295)
307 South Murray Street (38562)
Gainesboro, TN
(931) 268-0235
Fax: (931) 268-5678

JEFFERSON COUNTY
District 1, County #45
PO Box 490 (37725-0490)
L. C. Weaver Building
1050 South Highway 92 (37725)
Dandridge, TN
(423) 397-9401
Fax: (423) 397-1373

JOHNSON COUNTY
District 1, County #46
PO Box 912 (37683-0912)
150 East Main Street (37683-1610)
Mountain City, TN
(423) 727-7704
Fax: (423) 727-4404

KNOX COUNTY
District 2, County #47
State Office Building
531 Henley Street, Suite 310
Knoxville, TN 37902-2810
(423) 594-6713
Fax: (423) 594-6001

KNOX COUNTY B RANCH OFFICE
2700 Middlebrook Pike,
Suite 100
Knoxville, TN 37921-5602
(423) 594-6583
Fax: (423) 594-7045

LAKE COUNTY
District 7, County #48
760 Everett Street
Tiptonville, TN 38079-1608
(901) 253-7716
Fax: (901) 253-3326

LAUDERDALE COUNTY
District 7, County #49
417 South Washington Street
Ripley, TN 38063-9985
(901) 635-4141
Fax: (901) 221-0935

LAWRENCE COUNTY
District 5, County #50
PO Box 845 (38464-0845)
237 East Taylor Street (38464-3723)
Lawrenceburg, TN
(931) 766-1400
Fax: (931) 766-1461

LEWIS COUNTY
District 5, County #51
PO Box 99 (38462-0099)
200 Joe Avenue (38462-2002)
Hohenwald, TN
(931) 796-4971
Fax: (931) 796-4531

LINCOLN COUNTY
District 5, County #52
2221 Thornton Taylor Parkway
Fayetteville, TN 37334-3650
(931) 438-1925
Fax: (931) 438-1959

LOUDON COUNTY
District 1, County #53
301 South C Street
Lenoir City, TN 37771-2824
(423) 986-4751
Fax: (423) 988-8074

MACON COUNTY
District 3, County #54
PO Box 377 (37083-0377)
315 Highway 52E Bypass (37083)
Lafayette, TN
(615) 666-4041
Fax: (615) 666-3394

MADISON COUNTY
District 7, County #55
32 Conrad Drive
Jackson, TN 38305-2801
(901) 668-1041
Fax: (901) 661-6305

DISTRICT 7 JACKSON OFFICE
225 Martin Luther King Blvd.
Jackson, TN 38301
(901) 423-5850
Fax: (901) 423-5600
Fax: (901) 426-0563 "REHAB"

MARION COUNTY
District 3, County #56
PO Box 338 (37347-0338)
4926 Main Street (37347)
Jasper, TN
(423) 942-3481
Fax: (423) 942-8959

MARSHALL COUNTY
District 5, County #57
PO Box 1697 (37091-0697)
1204 Nashville Highway (37091-2222)
Lewisburg, TN
(931) 270-2234
Fax: (931) 270-2246

MAURY COUNTY
District 5, County #58
PO Box 800 (38402-0800)
209 Wayne Street (38401-4526)
Columbia, TN
(931) 380-2552
Fax: (931) 380-3396

DISTRICT 5 C OLUMBIA OFFICE
PO Box 239 (38402-0239) "FA"
PO Box 457 (38402-0457) "REHAB"
209 Wayne Street (38401-4526)
Columbia, TN
(931) 380-2568

MCMINN COUNTY
District 3, County #64
320 White Street, North
Athens, TN 37303-3504
(423) 744-2800
Fax: (423) 744-2596

MCNAIRY COUNTY
District 7, County #65
855 East Poplar Street
Selmer, TN 38375-1832
(901) 645-7994
Fax: (901) 645-8488

MEIGS COUNTY
District 3, County #59
PO Box 98 (37322-0098)
217 Highway 58, North (37322)
Decatur, TN
(423) 334-5787
Fax: (423) 334-1250

MONROE COUNTY
District 1, County #60
PO Box 188 (37354-0188)
876 Englewood Road (37354)
Madisonville, TN
(423) 442-7403
Fax: (423) 442-7408

MONTGOMERY COUNTY
District 5, County #61
350 Pageant Lane, Suite 301
Clarksville, TN 37040-3854
(931) 648-5500
Fax: (931) 572-1666

MOORE COUNTY
District 5, County #62
PO Box 202 (37352-0202)
2 Main Street (37352-9701)
Lynchburg, TN
(931) 759-7181
Fax: (931) 759-5917

MORGAN COUNTY
District 1, County #63
PO Box 344 (37887-0344)
Bardill Bldg., 830 Main Street (37887)
Wartburg, TN
(423) 346-6237
Fax: (423) 346-2831

OBION COUNTY
District 7, County #66
PO Box 428 (38261-0428)
1416 Stad Avenue (38261-5542)
Union City, TN
(901) 884-2603
Fax: (901) 884-2660

VERTON COUNTY
District 3, County #67
616 Church Street, North
Livingston, TN 38570-1199
(931) 823-5695
Fax: (931) 823-1499

PERRY COUNTY
District 5., County #68
PO Box 902 (37096-0902)
106 West Main Street (37096)
Linden, TN
(931) 589-2193
Fax: (931) 589-3641

PICKETT COUNTY
District 3, County #69
PO Box 400 (38549-0400)
8816 Highway 111 (38549)
Byrdstown, TN
(931) 864-3153
Fax: (931) 864-7156

POLK COUNTY
District 3, County #70
PO Box 160 (37307-0160)
7118 Highway 411, Suite 101 (37307)
Benton, TN
(423) 338-5332
Fax: (423) 338-0979

PUTNAM COUNTY
District 3, County #71
269-E South Willow Avenue
Cookeville, TN 38501-3110
(931) 528-7487
Fax: (931) 528-7450

Cookeville District 3 Office
444 Neal Street, East
Cookeville, TN 38501-4027
(931) 528-2591
Fax: (931) 528-9058

RHEA COUNTY
District 3, County #72
PO Box 70 (37321-0070)
224 4th Avenue, Suite 102 (37321)
Dayton, TN
(423) 775-2681
Fax: (423) 570-0534

ROANE COUNTY
District 1, County #73
PO Box 606 (37763-0606)
315 Race Street, East (37763-2828)
Kingston, TN
(423) 376-3491
Fax: (423) 717-1057

ROANE COUNTY REHAB. OFFICE
Harriman Occupational High School
PO Box 949
Harriman, TN 37748
(423) 882-1475

ROBERTSON COUNTY
District 5, County #74
809 Mabel Street
Springfield, TN 37172-2924
(615) 382-2402
Fax: (615) 382-3135

RUTHERFORD COUNTY
District 5, County #75
1711B Old Fort Parkway (37129)
Murfreesboro, TN
(615) 898-7000
Fax: (615) 848-7075

SCOTT COUNTY
District 1, County #76
PO Box 38 (37756-0038)
104 Fire Hall Drive (37756)
Huntsville, TN
(423) 663-2821
Fax: (423) 663-4095

SEQUATCHIE COUNTY
District 3, County #77
PO Box 848 (37327-0848)
108 Old York Highway East (37327-4121)
Dunlap, TN
(423) 949-4621
Fax: (423) 949-4868

SEVIER COUNTY
District 1, County #78
815 Dolly Parton Parkway
Sevierville, TN 37862-3698
(423) 429-7005
Fax: (423) 429-7051

SHELBY COUNTY
District 8, County #79
170 North Main Street
Memphis, TN 38103-1820
(901) 543-7351
Fax: (901) 543-6084
Fax: (901) 534-6036 "REHAB"

WELLES BRANCH OFFICE
3360 South 3rd Street
Memphis, TN 38109-2944
(901) 344-3650
Fax: (901) 344-3648

NORTH BRANCH OFFICE
3230 Jackson Avenue
Memphis, TN 38122-1011
(901) 320-7599
Fax: (901) 320-7335

MEMPHIS WORKS
4189 Leroy
Memphis, TN 38108

HURT VILLAGE
570 North 7th
Apartment E
Memphis, TN 38105
(901) 525-1514

SHELBY RESIDENTIAL & VOCATIONAL SVC SOUTH
1455 Poplar, 2nd Floor
Memphis, TN
(901) 276-2520

PARTNERS IN PLACEMENTS
3485 Poplar Avenue, Suite 205
Memphis, TN 38111

MEMPHIS GOODWILL INDUSTRIES, INC.
2605 Chelsea Avenue
Memphis, TN 38108
(901) 323-6221, Ext. 212

SMITH COUNTY
District 3, County #80
25 Dixon Springs Highway
Carthage, TN 37030-1093
(615) 735-9740
Fax: (615) 735-1776

STEWART COUNTY
District 5, County #81
PO Box 370 (37058-0370)
1011 Spring Street (37058-3302)
Dover, TN
(931) 232-5304
Fax: (931) 232-2349

SULLIVAN COUNTY
District 1, Cty #82
PO Box 1511 (37662-1511)
201 Cherokee Street (37660-4309)
Kingsport, TN
(423) 224-1900
Fax: (423) 224-1974

SULLIVAN BRANCH OFFICE
PO Box 3965 (37625-3965)
2305 Volunteer Parkway (37625)
Bristol, TN
(615) 968-9133
Fax: (615) 968-6775

COMMUNITY HEALTH AGENCY
441 Clay Street
Kingsport, TN 37660
(615) 246-7225

SUMNER COUNTY
District 5, County #83
PO Box 1687 (37066-1687)
447 East Broadway (37066-2322)
Gallatin, TN
(615) 451-5814
Fax: (615) 451-6394

TIPTON COUNTY
District 7, County #84
724 Highway 51, North (38019-2037)
Covington, TN
(901) 475-2505
Fax: (901) 475-2617

TROUSDALE COUNTY
District 5, County #85
PO Box 53 (37074-0053)
205 East Main Street (37074-1705)
Hartsville, TN
(615) 374-3513
Fax: (615) 374-3237

UNICOI COUNTY
District 1, County #86
724 Ohio Avenue
Erwin, TN 37650
(423) 743-3166
Fax: (423) 743-1122

UNION COUNTY
District 1, County #87
PO Box 40 (37807-0040)
701 Main Street (37807)
Maynardville, TN
(423) 992-5802
Fax: (423) 992-7250

VAN BUREN COUNTY
District 3, County #88
PO Box 361 (38585-0361)
Spring Street (38585-9757)
Spencer, TN
(931) 946-2437
Fax: (931) 946-7804

WARREN COUNTY
District 3, County #89
1200 Belmont Drive
McMinnville, TN 37110-8652
(931) 473-9633
Fax: (931) 473-3796

WASHINGTON COUNTY
District 1, County #90
PO Box 1358 (37605-1358)
103 Walnut Street, East (37601-6847)
Johnson City, TN
(423) 929-0171
Fax: (423) 434-6974

DISTRICT 1 OFFICE
PO Box 2120 (37604)
213 Maple Street, West (37601)
Johnson City, TN
(423) 929-9142

WASHINGTON REHAB OFFICE
PO Box 2120
905 Buffalo Street
Johnson City, TN 37604
(423) 926-3178
Fax: (423) 929-2944

WAYNE COUNTY
District 5, County #91
PO Box 687 (38485-0687)
212 South High Street (38485-2616)
Waynesboro, TN
(615) 722-3431
Fax: (615) 722-7881

WEAKLEY COUNTY
District 7, County #92
PO Box 729 (38225-0729)
8616 Highway 22 (38225-2308)
Dresden, TN
(901) 364-2366
Fax: (901) 364-2348

WHITE COUNTY
District 3, County #93
826 Valley View Drive
Sparta, TN 38583-1233
(931) 738-8256
Fax: (931) 738-3763

WILLIAMSON COUNTY
District 5, County #94
PO Box 680909 (37068-0909)
203-B. Beasley Drive (37064-3907)
Franklin, TN
(615) 790-5502
Fax: (615) 790-5652

WILSON COUNTY
District 5, County #95
PO Box 806 (37088-0806)
712 North Cumberland (37088-2312)
Lebanon, TN
(615) 443-2751
Fax: (615) 443-2761

TEXAS DEPARTMENT OF HUMAN SERVICES REGION I AND III:

AMARILLO
3501-L West 45th Street
PO Box 3700
Amarillo, TX 79116-3700
(806) 352-5005
Fax: (806) 356-3180
TDD: (806) 356-3101

BORGER
100 Veta Street
PO Box 3309
Borger, TX 79007-3309
(806) 273-7517
Fax: (806) 274-5028

BROWNFIELD
101 North Avenue D
PO Box 1072
Brownfield, TX 79316-1072
(806) 637-8576
Fax: (806) 637-7181

CHILDRESS
801 Commerce Street
PO Box 76
Childress, TX 79201
(940) 937-6301
Fax: (940) 937-6398

CLARENDON
911 East 2nd Street
PO Box 1109
Clarendon, TX 79226-1109
(806) 874-3595
Fax: (806) 874-5119

DIMMITT
204 South East 3rd Street
PO Box 517
Dimmitt, TX 79027-0517
(806) 647-4181
Fax: (806) 647-4578

DUMAS
810 Dumas Avenue
Dumas, TX 79029-4399
(806) 935-6837
Fax: (806) 935-5855

HEREFORD
212 North 25 Mile Avenue
Hereford, TX 79045-60169
(806) 364-6841
Fax: (806) 363-8629

LEVELLAND
904 8th Street
PO Box 817
Levelland, TX 79336-3599
(806) 894-9606
Fax: (806) 897-4248

LITTLEFIELD
210 Marshall Howard Blvd.
PO Box 710
Littlefield, TX 79339
(806) 385-4416
Fax: (806) 385-7902

LUBBOCK
5806 34th Street
PO Box 10528
Lubbock, TX 79408-3528
(806) 797-8870
Fax: (806) 791-7590
TDD: (806) 791-7518

PAMPA
1509 North Banks
Pampa, TX 79065-4147
(806) 665-1863
Fax: (806) 663-5353

PLAINVIEW
2907 West 7th Street
Plainview, TX 79072-6731
(806) 293-5193
Fax: (806) 296-3165

POST
US 84 South
PO Box 100
Post, TX 79356-0100
(806) 495-2881
Fax: (806) 495-2419

SHAMROCK
113 West 2nd Street
Shamrock, TX 79079-2292
(806) 256-2164
Fax: (806) 256-2008

REGION II AND IX:

ABILENE
317 Pecan
PO Box 6635
Abilene, TX 79608-6635
(915) 673-5217

ANDREWS
801 North Main
Andrews, TX 79714-8133
(915) 523-2118

ANSON
1301 South Commercial
PO Box 31
Anson, TX 79501-0031
(915) 823-3285

BAIRD
124 West 4th Street
Baird, TX 79504
(915) 854-1257

BALLINGER
614 Strong
PO Box 347
Ballinger, TX 76821
(915) 365-2564

BIG LAKE
300 Plaza
PO Box 961
Big Lake, TX 76932
(915) 884-3245

BIG SPRING
501 Birdwell Lane
Suite 28E
Big Spring, TX 79720
(915) 263-9625

BOWIE
601 East Decatur
Bowie, TX 76230
(915) 872-1196

BRADY
302 West Lockhart
PO Box 829
Brady, TX 76825
(915) 597-0751

BRECKENRIDGE
2802 West Walker
PO Box 1554
Breckenridge, TX 76424
(254) 559-8294

BROWNWOOD
301 Main
Brownwood, TX 76801
(915) 646-0541

COLEMAN
114 Needham
PO Box 999
Coleman, TX 76834
(915) 625-4183

COLORADO CITY
440 East 2nd Street
Colorado City, TX 79512
(915) 728-2618

COMANCHE
400 Industrial
PO Box 493
Comanche, TX 76442
(915) 356-2554

CRANE
1212 South Alford
Crane, TX 79731
(915) 558-7145

EASTLAND
1331 East Main
Eastland, TX 76448
(254) 629-3317

FORT STOCKTON
108 West Walter
PO Box 550
Fort Stockton, TX 79735
(915) 336-9745

GRAHAM
1202 Packing House Road
Graham, TX 76450
(940) 549-1371

HASKELL
420 North First Street
PO Box 817
Haskell, TX 79521
(940) 864-2694

HENRIETTA
1101 North Bridge
Henrietta, TX 76365
(940) 538-5201

JACKSBORO
100 North Main
PO Box B
Jacksboro, TX 76458
(940) 567-2471

JUNCTION
1003 College Drive
PO Box 326
Junction, TX 76849-0326
(915) 446-2920

KERMIT
401 South Pine
Kermit, TX 79745
(915) 586-3451

KNOX CITY
606 East Main
PO Box 368
Knox City, TX 79529
(940) 658-3524

LAMESA
701 South Bryan
Lamesa, TX 79331
(806) 872-5481

MENARD
104 San Saba
PO Box 548
Menard, TX 76859
(915) 396-4505

MIDLAND
901 West Wall
Third Floor
Midland, TX 79701
(915) 686-2313
(915) 686-2312

MONAHANS
110 West B Street
Monahans, TX 79756
(915) 943-6745

NOCONA
910 West Highway 82
PO Box 418
Nocona, TX 76255
(940) 825-3796

ODESSA
3016 Kermit Highway
Odessa, TX 79764
(915) 334-5100

ODESSA
2330 West 10th
Odessa, TX 79762
(915) 335-3600

OLNEY
210 West Main
PO Box 68
Olney, TX 76374
(940) 564-2396

OZONA
616 Avenue H
PO Box 1736
Ozona, TX 76943
(915) 392-5131

PADUCAH
724 9th Street
PO Box 888
Paducah, TX 79248
(806) 492-3576

PECOS
1705 West 4th Street
Pecos, TX 79772
(915) 445-5487

QUANAH
300 Main Street
PO Box 449
Quanah, TX 79252
(940) 663-6307

ROBY
107 East North 1st
PO Box 400
Roby, TX 79543
(915) 776-2234

SAN ANGELO
622 South Oakes
Suite E-1
San Angelo, TX 76903
(915) 659-7900

SEMINOLE
600 Hobbs Highway
Seminole, TX 79360
(915) 758-9463

SEYMOUR
115 West Morris
PO Box 792
Seymour, TX 76380
(940) 888-3536

SNYDER
3409 Snyder Shopping Center
PO Box 1037
Snyder, TX 79550
(915) 573-1161

SONORA
1004 Eaton
Suite A
Sonora, TX 76950
(915) 387-5066

STANTON
310 North Street Peter
PO Box 930
Stanton, TX 79782
(915) 756-2805

SWEETWATER
3rd Floor, 100 East 3rd
PO Box 1459
Sweetwater, TX 79556
(915) 235-8401

VERNON
1531 Cumberland
Vernon, TX 76384
(940) 552-6238

WICHITA FALLS
600 Scott Street
Wichita Falls, TX 76301
(940) 766-3371

WINTERS
110 South Main
Suite 107
Winters, TX 79567
(915) 754-5469

REGION IV:

ATHENS
101 West Bakers Street
Athens, TX 75751-4409
(903) 675-9141

ATHENS
115 South Murchison
Athens, TX 75751-2662
(903) 675-5631

ATLANTA
323 East Thomas
Atlanta, TX 75551-2836
(903) 796-2861

CANTON
555 West Highway 2443
Canton, TX 75103-2113
(903) 567-4147

CARTHAGE
1412 South Adams
Carthage, TX 75633-3242
(903) 693-7817

CLARKSVILLE
308 North Cedar
PO Box 905
Clarksville, TX 75426-3017

COOPER
1280 West Dallas
Rt. 2, PO Box 313
Cooper, TX 75432-9736
(903) 395-2154

DAINGERFIELD
603 Ward Street
Dangerfield, TX 75638-1547
(903) 645-2283

DEKALB
101 North East Houston
Dekalb, TX 75559-1430
(903) 667-2504

EMORY
120 South Texas Street
Alexander Bldg./ TX SH 19
PO Box 86
Emory, TX 75440-0086
(903) 473-2293

GILMER
324 Yapaco Street
Gilmer, TX 75644-2360
(903) 843-5049

GLADEWATER
309 West Gregg
Gladewater, TX 75647-2157
(903) 845-2246

HENDERSON
1400 Wilson Street
Henderson, TX 75652-6038
(903) 657-5508

JACKSONVILLE
502 East Pine
Jacksonville, TX 5766-4566
(903) 586-7626

JEFFERSON
1113 North Walcott
Jefferson, TX 75657-1041
(903) 665-3926

KILGORE
1501 Pentecost
Kilgore, TX 75662-5634
(903) 984-0581

LINDEN
213 Highway 8 North
Linden, TX 75563-9514
(903) 756-5551

LONGVIEW
1750 North Eastman
Longview, TX 75601-3347
(903) 753-0083

MARSHALL
4105 Victory Drive
Marshall, TX 75672-4751
(903) 938-7751

MINEOLA
714 Greenville Hwy.
Mineola, TX 75773-1010
(903) 569-5368

MT. PLEASANT
303 East 11th Street
Mt. Pleasant, TX 75455-2598
(903) 572-3483

MT. VERNON
502 East Main
Mt. Vernon, TX 75457-2507
(903) 537-4541

NEW BOSTON
912 South Merrill
New Boston, TX 75570-3512
(903) 628-5513

PALESTINE
811 North Mallard
Palestine, TX 75801-2493
(903) 729-0174

PARIS
400 West Sherman Street
Paris, TX 75460-5646
(903) 785-7541

PITTSBURG
211 Mill Street
Pittsburg, TX 75686-1315
(903) 856-3678

QUITMAN
305 West Goodwin Street
Quitman, TX 75783-2427
(903) 763-2275

RUSK
201 West First
Rusk, TX 75785-1203
(903) 683-5473

SULPHUR SPRINGS
1400 College Street
Sulphur Springs, TX 75482-3431
(903) 885-9561

TEXARKANA
3115 South Lake Drive, Suite 120
Liberty Square Mall
Texarkana, TX 75501-7907
(903) 791-6400

TYLER
3303 Mineola Highway
Tyler, TX 75702-1126
(903) 595-4841

WINNSBORO
1001 East Coke Road
Winnsboro, TX 75494-3536
(903) 342-5663

REGION V:

BEAUMONT
285 Liberty
PO Box 4906
Beaumont, TX 77704-4906
(409) 981-5920
A&D: 77701, 77702, 77703, 77705, 77706, 77707, 77708, 77709, 77710,
77713, 77613, 77720, 77726, 77376
CSS: 77701, 77702, 77703, 77705, 77706, 77707, 77708, 77709, 77710,
77613, 77720, 77726, 77722, 77622, 77627, 77629, 77665

BEAUMONT
3420 Fannin
Suite 220
Beaumont, TX 77701-3803
(409) 833-0072

BUNA
South East Corner Camelia & Commerce
PO Box 1138
Buna, TX 77612-1138
(409) 994-5926
CSS: 77612, 77614, 77615, 77662, 75956, 77632, 77630

CENTER
108 Austin
PO Box 1689
Center, TX 75935-1689
(409) 598-6368
Zip Code: 73935, 75954, 75972, 75973, 75974, 75975

COLDSPRING
County Courthouse
PO Box 10
Coldspring, TX 77331-0010
(409) 653-4391
A&D: 77331, 77327, 77358, 77359
CSS: 77331, 77378, 77371, 77364,77359, 77358, 77327

CORRIGAN
209 West Ben Franklin
Corrigan, TX 75939-2003
(409) 398-4188
A&D: 77351, 77360, 77335, 77364, 77326, 77332, 75939, 77350, 75936, 75934, 75930, 77350
CSS: 75939, 77350, 75936, 75934, 75960, 75965, 77351

CROCKETT
111 NW Loop 304
PO Box 959
Crockett, TX 75835-0959
(409) 544-2123
A&D: 75835, 75851, 75849, 75847, 75844, 75858, 75856, 75830

GROVETON
Rock Building
PO Box 40
Groveton, TX 75845-0040
(409) 642-1134
A&D: 75926, 75854, 75856, 75862, 75865
CSS: 75845, 75360, 75865, 75851, 75856, 75926, 75847, 75862, 75834

HEMPHILL
201 Pineland
PO Box 1927
Hemphill, TX 75948-1927
(409) 787-3871
A&D: 75930, 75931, 75941, 75945, 75946, 75947, 75948, 75949, 75959, 75968, 75969, 75973
CSS: 75948, 75931, 75930, 75947, 75959, 75968, 75972

JASPER
720 South Wheeler
Jasper, TX 75951-4544
(409) 383-5510
A&D: 75951, 75931, 75956, 77364, 77371, 77378, 75957, 75966, 75977, 75928, 75932
CSS: 75951, 75931, 75956, 75966

KIRBYVILLE
314 North Herndon
PO Box 900
Kirbyville, TX 75956-0971
(409) 423-4612
Zip Code: 75951, 75956, 75933, 75957
CSS: 75956, 75933, 75957

KOUNTZE
County Courthouse Annex
PO Box 250
Kountze, TX 77625-0250
(409) 246-3472
AD: 77711, 77625, 77656, 77657, 77659, 77663, 75956, 77616, 77585
CSS: 77519, 77663, 77585, 77376, 77625

LIVINGSTON
1102 M.L.K.
Suite A
Livingston, TX 77351-2644
(409) 327-3472
A&D: 77369, 77327, 77358, 77378
CSS: 77351, 77335, 77326, 77369, 77360, 77332, 77350

LUFKIN
210 Christie Street
Lufkin, TX 75901-0508
(936) 632-7708
A&D: 75901, 75902, 75903, 75904, 75915, 75941, 75949, 75969, 75980
CSS: 75901, 75902, 75903, 75904, 75915, 75969, 75941, 75949, 75980

NACOGDOCHES
320 North Street
PO Box 631334
Nacogdoches, TX 75963-1334
(936) 569-1779
Zip Code: 75961, 75962, 75963, 75964, 75760, 75943, 75978, 75937, 75946, 75944, 75958, 75788

NACOGDOCHES
204 Mims Street
Nacogdoches, TX 75961-4578
(936) 560-3058

NEWTON
Old Hospital
PO Box 568
Newton, TX 75966-0568
(409) 379-3451
A&D: 75956, 75966, 75977, 75933, 75932, 75932, 75928

ORANGE
308 Cypress
Orange, TX 77630-5198
(409) 883-3085
A&D: 77630, 77631, 77632, 77614, 77611, 77639, 77626, 77613

PORT ARTHUR
5860 9th Avenue
PO Box 2606
Port Arthur, TX 77643-2606
(409) 962-2001
A&D: 77640, 77641, 77642, 77643, 77619, 77651, 77627, 77655
CSS: 77619, 77627, 77640, 77641, 77643, 77651, 77655

SAN AUGUSTINE
County Courthouse
PO Box 516
San Augustine, TX 75972-0516
(409) 275-3458
A&D: 75922, 75930, 75973, 75937, 75972
CSS: 75972, 75930, 75929, 75935, 75947

SILSBEE
1215 Highway 327 East
Silsbee, TX 77656-5119
(409) 385-5290
A&D: 77374, 77650, 77633, 77369, 77656, 77376, 77625, 77567, 77585, 77659, 77519, 77657, 77757, 77612, 77615
CSS: 77519, 77663, 77585, 77625, 77376

TRINITY
832 South Robb
PO Box 2330
Trinity, TX 75862
(409) 594-6380
A&D: 75862, 75845, 75926, 75865, 75856,
CSS: 75862, 77367

VIDOR
1091 North Main
Suite B
Vidor, TX 77662-4839
(409) 769-1631
A&D: 77662, 77611, 77639

WOODVILLE
930 North Magnolia
PO Box 368
Woodville, TX 75979-0368
(409) 283-3765
A&D: 75938, 75979, 75942, 77616, 77624, 77660, 77663, 77664,
75979, 77970
CSS: 75979, 75942, 77660,75936, 77616, 77664, 75938, 77624,
77656, 75951

REGION VI:

ALVIN
3403 Mustang Road
Alvin, TX 77511
(281) 331-0790
Zip code: 77511, 77512, 77577, 77578, 77583, 77584, 77588

ANAHUAC
204 North Texas Avenue
Anahuac, TX 77514
(409) 267-3125
TDD: (409) 267-4383
Zip Code: 77514, 77520 (Chambers), 77521(Chambers), 77535, 77560,
77575, 77579, 77580, 77597, 77661, 77665

ANGLETON
UTMB Regional Maternal & Child Health Center
1108 East Mulberry
Angleton, TX 77515
(979) 849-0739
TDD: (979) 849-0739

BAY CITY
Matagorda County Hospital
1115 Avenue G
Bay City, TX 77414
(979) 245-5201
Zip Code: 77414, 77456, 77756

BAY CITY
1605 7th Street
Bay City, TX 77414
(979) 244-1662
Zip Code: 77404, 77414, 77415, 77419, 77420, 77428, 77431, 77432,

BAYTOWN
1300 South Highway 146
Baytown, TX 77520
(281) 427-9480
TDD: (281) 593-7212 x257
Zip Code: 77520 (Harris Co.),77521 (Harris Co.)

BAYTOWN
Baycoast Medical Center
1700 James Bowie Dr.
Baytown, TX 77522
(281) 420-6473
TDD: (281) 420-6473

BELLVILLE
800 East Wendt
Bellville, TX 77418
(409) 865-9164
Zip Code: 77418, 77452, 77473, 77474, 77485, 78931, 78933, 78944, 78954

BROOKSHIRE
535 FM 359 South
PO Box 367
Brookshire, TX 77423
(281) 375-5176
Zip Code: 77423,77449,77450,77466,77492,77493,77494

CLEVELAND
807 East Hanson
Cleveland, TX 77327
(281) 592-0531
TDD: (281) 593-7212
Zip Code: 77327,77328,77357,77368,77369,77372

CLUTE
794 South Brazosport Blvd.
Clute, TX 77531
(409) 265-1291
TDD: (409) 266-3505
Zip Codes: 77422,77486,77515,77516,77534,77531,77541,77566

COLUMBUS
1460 Walnut
Columbus, TX 78934
(409) 732-6231
Zip Codes: 77412, 77434, 77442, 77460, 77470, 77475, 78934, 78935, 78943, 78950, 78951, 78962

CONROE
108 Commercial Circle
Conroe, TX 77304
(409) 539-1161
TDD: (409) 760-4722
Zip Codes: 77301, 77302, 77303, 77304, 77305, 77306, 77327, 77333, 77339, 77356, 77357, 77365, 77372, 77378, 77380, 77381, 77382, 77384, 77385, 77386, 77390

CONROE
Columbia Conroe Regional Medical Center
500 Medical Center Blvd
Suite 155
Conroe, TX 77304
(936) 539-7095
TDD: (936) 539-7095
Zip Codes: 77301, 77302, 77303, 77304, 77305, 77339, 77333, 77386, 77333, 77386, 77385, 77381, 77389, 77384, 77372, 77327, 77365

CONROE
UTMB Regional Maternal & Child Health Clinic
701 East Davis
Conroe, TX 77301
(936) 525-2894
TDD: (936) 525-2894

CROSBY
6500 North Main
Crosby, TX 77532
(281) 328-6613
TDD: (281) 328-6613
Zip Codes: 77336,77532,77692

DICKINSON
UTMB Maternal & Child Health Center
2727 44th Street
Dickinson, TX 77539
(281) 534-2576

DICKINSON
215 Tanglewood
Dickinson, TX 77539
(281) 337-5402
(409) 945-4476 x236 (TDD)
TDD: (281) 534-2576
Zip Codes: 77510, 77511, 77517, 77518, 77539, 77546, 77563, 77565, 77573, 77586

GALVESTON
University of Texas Medical Branch UHC
301 University Ave, Room 1.606
Galveston, TX 77555-1393
(409) 772-7525
TDD: (409) 772-7525
Zip Codes: 77550,77551,77553,77554

GALVESTON
301 University Route 0859
Galveston, TX 77550
(409) 747-4935
Zip Codes: 77550,77551,77553,77554

GALVESTON
123 Rosenberg, #500
Galveston, TX 77550
(409) 763-0277
TDD: (409) 747-7757
Zip Codes: 77550,77551,77552,77553,77554,77617,77623,77650

GALVESTON
University of Texas Medical Branch PC Pavilion
400 Harborside Drive
Galveston, TX 77550
(409) 747-4936
Zip Codes: 77550,77551,77553,77554

HEMPSTEAD
1739 13th Street
Hempstead, TX 77445
(409) 826-8211
TDD: (409) 826-8211
Zip Codes: 77363,77445,77446,77447,77484

HOUSTON
9111 Eastex Freeway
Houston, TX 77093
(713) 691-0033
TDD: (713) 696-5130
Zip Codes: 77016,77026,77028,77044,77049,77050,77078

HOUSTON
Southwest Community Health Center
6441 High Star
Houston, TX 77074
(713) 779-6400
TDD: (713) 746-6400 x263

HOUSTON
9460 Harwin
Houston, TX 77036
(713) 783-0828
TDD: (713) 268-1481
Zip Codes: 77031,77072,77074,77099

HOUSTON
9450 Harwin
Houston, TX 77036
(713) 266-5535
TDD: (713) 268-1481
Zip Codes: 77036,77046,77081,77083,77411,77477,77478

HOUSTON
1100 Greens Parkway
Houston, TX 77067
(281) 874-0048
TDD: (281) 775-7960
Zip Codes: 77014, 77040, 77041, 77060, 77064, 77065, 77066, 77067, 77068, 77069, 77070, 77086, 77090, 77095, 77337, 77389, 77429, 77433

HOUSTON
10060 Fuqua
Houston, TX 77089
(713) 946-6861
TDD: (713) 948-7909
Zip Codes: 77034, 77058, 77059, 77061, 77062, 77075, 77089, 77209, 77504, 77505, 77507, 77581, 77587, 77598

HOUSTON
UTHSC-Houston
7000 Fannin
Suite 2340
Houston, TX 77030
(713) 500-3483

HOUSTON
Texas Children's Hospital
6621 Fannin
Houston, TX 77030
(713) 770-5523
TDD: (713) 770-5523

HOUSTON
Columbia Sunbelt Medical Center
13111 I-10 East
Houston, TX 77015
(713) 457-8292

HOUSTON
Harris County Hospital District/ SW Reg. Center
6654 Hornwood
Houston, TX 77074
(713) 995-3551
TDD: (713) 995-3531

HOUSTON
1320 East 40th
Houston, TX 77022
(713) 696-8025

HOUSTON
Columbia Bellaire Medical Center
5314 Dashwood
Houston, TX 77081
(713) 512-1426
TDD: (713) 667-0079

HOUSTON
13838 Buffalo Speedway
Houston, TX 77045
(713) 433-3145
TDD: (713) 434-3145
Zip Codes: 77035, 77045, 77047, 77048, 77053, 77054, 77071, 77085, 77096

HOUSTON
1504 Ben Taub Loop
Houston, TX 77030
(713) 678-3202
TDD: (713) 852-3957

HOUSTON
Sharpstown General Hospital
6700 Bellaire Boulevard
Houston, TX 77074
(713) 774-7611
TDD: (713) 778-2621

HOUSTON
Harris County Hospital District
2525 Holly Hall
Houston, TX 77054
(713) 746-6464
TDD: (713) 746-6464

HOUSTON
Hermann Hospital
6411 Fannin
Houston, TX 77030
(713) 704-3405
TDD: (713) 704-3405

HOUSTON
State of Texas Building
5425 Polk Street
Houston, TX 77023
(713) 767-2000
TDD: (713) 767-2438

HOUSTON
12121 Westheimer
Houston, TX 77077
(713) 597-5200
TDD: (281) 597-5204
Zip Codes: 77024, 77042, 77043, 77056, 77057, 77063, 77077, 77079, 77080, 77082, 77084, 77094, 77413

HOUSTON
2110 Telephone Road
Houston, TX 77023
(713) 921-5108
TDD: (713) 967-7565
Zip Codes: 77003, 77006, 77011, 77012, 77017, 77019, 77020, 77023, 77029, 77087, 77547

HOUSTON
MD Anderson Hospital
1515 Holcombe Blvd
Houston, TX 77030
(713) 791-1005
TDD: (713) 792-6144

HOUSTON
6118 Scott
Houston, TX 77021
(713) 748-8450
TDD: (713) 746-3091
Zip Codes: 77001, 77002, 77004, 77005, 77021, 77025, 77030, 77033,
77051, 77052, 77401

HOUSTON
Columbia North Houston Medical Center
233 North Parker
Houston, TX 77076
(713) 697-2831

HOUSTON
1440 North Loop
Houston, TX 77009
(713) 863-9864
TDD: (713) 803-1995
Zip Codes: 77007,77008,77009,77010,77027,77055,77098

HOUSTON
Harris County Hospital District/ N Loop E Reg Cen
7100 N Loop East
Suite A-16
Houston, TX 77028
(713) 678-1020
TDD: (713) 678-1020

HOUSTON
7333 North Freeway
Houston, TX 77076
(713) 691-7711
TDD: (713) 696-1697
Zip Codes: 77018,77022,77088,77091

HOUSTON
2711 Little York
Houston, TX 77093
(713) 699-1098
TDD: (713) 696-7218

HOUSTON
Harris County Hospital/ S Loop Reg. Center
5959 Long Drive
Houston, TX 77087
(713) 845-3800
TDD: (713) 845-3827
Zip Codes: 77032,77037,77038,77039,77076,77092,77093

HOUSTON
Street Joseph Hospital
1919 Labranch
Houston, TX 77002
(713) 657-7329
TDD: (713) 756-5927

HOUSTON
Lyndon B. Johnson Hospital
5656 Kelly
Houston, TX 77026
(713) 636-5378

HOUSTON
Jacinto Plaza, Bldg 1
10202 I-10 East
Houston, TX 77029
(713) 673-6347
TDD: (713) 671-8833
Zip Codes: 77013,77015,77026,77029,77530,77547

HOUSTON
Ben Taub Hospital
1504 Taub Loop
Houston, TX 77030
(713) 793-2254

HUMBLE
3000 Wilson Road
Humble, TX 77396
(281) 446-0209
Zip Codes: 77073, 77205, 77338, 77345, 77346, 77347, 77357, 77365, 77373, 77383, 77388, 77396

HUNTSVILLE
1401 Avenue N
Huntsville, TX 77340
(936) 291-2164
Zip Codes: 77334,77340,77341,77358,77367

HUNTSVILLE
UTMB Huntsville Clinic
1217 Avenue North
Huntsville, TX 77340
(936) 295-7474
TDD: (936) 295-7474

LA PORTE
1003 South Broadway
La Porte, TX 77571
(281) 470-8355
Zip Codes: 77536,77571,77586

LIBERTY
2800 Beaumont Ave
Liberty, TX 77575
(409) 336-7283
TDD: (409) 336-4811
Zip Codes: 77533,77535,77536,77538,77561,77564,77575,77582

NEW CANEY
New Caney UTMB Clinic
Highway 59
Courthouse Annex
New Caney, TX 77357
(281) 354-5773
TDD: (281) 557-8966

PASADENA
SE Clinic/ Pasadena UTMB Clinic
3737 Red Bluff RD
Pasadena, TX 77503
(713) 740-5010
TDD: (713) 740-5024

PASADENA
Memorial Hospital Pasadena
906 East Southmore
Pasadena, TX 77502
(713) 477-0411

PASADENA
Columbia Bayshore Medical Center
4000 Spencer Highway
Pasadena, TX 77506
(713) 948-1156
TDD: (713) 359-1156

PASADENA
Strawberry Clinic
1029 Strawberry
Pasadena, TX 77502
(713) 740-8172
TDD: (713) 982-5936

PASADENA
2702 Cherrybrook
Pasadena, TX 77502
(713) 947-8130
TDD: (713) 948-2033
Zip Codes: 77501,77502,77503,77506,77508

PEARLAND
Pasadena UTMB Pearland Clinic
4616 West Broadway Suite F
Pearland, TX 77581
(409) 772-5074
TDD: (281) 485-0165

RICHMOND
Fort Bend Family Health Center
400 Austin Street
Richmond, TX 77469
(281) 342-0500
TDD: (281) 341-2900 x116

ROSENBERG
117 Lane Drive
Rosenberg, TX 77471
(281) 342-8651
TDD: (281) 344-3456
Zip Codes: 77031, 77045, 77053, 77071, 77083, 77099, 77417, 77421, 77430, 77441, 77444, 77451, 77459, 77461, 77464, 77469, 77471, 77476, 77477, 77478, 77479, 77481, 77485, 77489, 77545, 77583

STAFFORD
Fort Bend Family Health Center New Hope Clinic
10435 Greenbough
Suite 300
Stafford, TX 77477
(281) 261-0182
TDD: (281) 261-7326 x111

STAFFORD
UTMB Regional Maternal & Child Health Center
2503 South Main
Stafford, TX 77477
(713) 261-7219
TDD: (281) 261-7219

SWEENEY
Sweeney Hospital District
305 North McKinney
Sweeney, TX 77480
(409) 548-3311
TDD: (281) 261-7219

TEXAS CITY
Columbia Mainland Medical Center
State Highway 3 @ FM 1764
Texas City, TX 77592
(409) 996-5000

TEXAS CITY
2000 Texas Avenue
Texas City, TX 77590
(409) 945-0317
TDD: (409) 945-0317
TWD (Handles last names beginning with L-Z)
Zip Codes: 77568,77590,77591,77592

TEXAS CITY
714 Loop 197
Texas City, TX 77590
(409) 948-1701
TDD: (409) 943-2844
TWD (Handles last names beginning with A-K)
Zip Codes: 77568,77590,77591,77592

TOMBALL
500 West Main
Tomball, TX 77375
(281) 351-0637
TDD: (281) 351-0637
Zip Codes: 77353,77354,77355,77362,77375,77379,77447

WHARTON
Columbia Gulf Coast Medical Center
1400 Highway Bypass
Wharton, TX 77488
(409) 282-6104

WHARTON
404 North Alabama Road
Wharton, TX 77488
(409) 532-5910
Zip Codes: 77420, 77432, 77434, 77435, 77436, 77437, 77443, 77448, 77453, 77454, 77455, 77462, 77467, 77468, 77488

WHARTON
UTMB Regional Maternal & Child Health Clinic
2407 Richmond
Wharton, TX 77488
(409) 532-0902
TDD: (409) 532-0902

REGION VII:

AUSTIN
1601 Rutherford Lane
Austin, TX 78754-5125
(512) 339-8868
TDD: (512) 876-6333

AUSTIN
1165 Airport Boulevard
Austin, TX 78702-3153
(512) 929-7330
TDD: (512) 919-7295

AUSTIN
724 Eberhart Lane
Austin, TX 78745-3938
(512) 445-0022
TDD: (512) 416-5299

AUSTIN
7901 Cameron Road
Building 1 & 2
Austin, TX 78754-3831
(512) 832-7745
TDD: (512) 832-7795

AUSTIN
10205 North Lamar
Austin, TX 78753-3658
(512) 834-0162
TDD: (512) 908-9697

BASTROP
3809 Loop 150 East
Bastrop, TX 78602-5013
(512) 321-3995
TDD: (512) 321-8162

BRENHAM
2505 Stone Hollow
Brenham, TX 77833-5631
(979) 836-7951
TDD: (979) 830-6190

BRYAN
3000 East Villa Maria
Bryan, TX 77803-5015
(979) 776-1510

BURNET
1004 Buchannan Drive
Suite 2
Burnet, TX 78611-2327
(512) 756-6071

CALDWELL
500 West Highway 21
Caldwell, TX 77836-1126
(409) 567-3283

CAMERON
605 West 4th
Cameron, TX 76520-2406
(254) 697-2353
TDD: (254) 697-6044

CENTERVILLE
East Highway 7
Centerville, TX 75833
(903) 536-2743

COPPERAS COVE
317 Casa Drive
Copperas Cove, TX 76522-3909
(254) 547-4286

ELGIN
218 South Main
Elgin, TX 78621-2942
(512) 285-9665

GATESVILLE
1409-A East Main
Gatesville, TX 76528-1668
(254) 865-7291

GEORGETOWN
601 Quail Valley Drive
Georgetown, TX 78626-8051
(512) 863-6581
TDD: (512) 868-9831

GIDDINGS
849 East Industry
Giddings, TX 78942-4301
(409) 542-3621

GOLDTHWAITE
2nd Floor County Courthouse
Goldthwaite, TX 76844
(915) 648-2710

HAMILTON
103 Parkhill
Hamilton, TX 76531-1542
(254) 386-4993

HARKER HEIGHTS
331 Indian Trail
Harker Heights, TX 76548-7207
(254) 690-7800
TDD: (254) 690-0002

HEARNE
101 Cedar
Hearne, TX 77859-2522
(409) 279-3446
TDD: (409) 279-5896

HILLSBORO
605 South Ivy
Hillsboro, TX 76645-3513
(254) 582-5321
TDD: (254) 582-0377

KILLEEN
315 East Street, Avenue D
Killeen, TX 76541-5240
(254) 519-4666
TDD: (254) 519-7563

LA GRANGE
228 North Main
La Grange, TX 78945-2234
(409) 968-3196
TDD: (409) 968-8396

LAMPASAS
204 Riverview
Lampasas, TX 76550
(512) 556-3629
TDD: (512) 556-4333

LLANO
Highway 71 East
Llano, TX 78643
(915) 247-3270

LOCKHART
1400 FM 20
Lockhart, TX 78644-3778
(512) 398-4541
TDD: (512) 398-9728

LULING
505 East Fannin
Luling, TX 78648-2325
(830) 875-5603

MADISONVILLE
300 West School Street
Suite 200
Madisonville, TX 77864-3279
(409) 348-2727

MARBLE FALLS
1200 Avenue K
Suite 100
Marble Falls, TX 78654-5017
(830) 693-5703
TDD: (830) 693-7893

MARLIN
211 Williams Street
Marlin, TX 76661-3026
(254) 883-3555
TDD: (254) 883-2904

MERIDIAN
401 South Hill Street
Meridian, TX 76665
(254) 435-2302

MEXIA
404 East Palestine
Mexia, TX 76667-2837
(254) 562-3861
TDD: (254) 562-7147

NAVASOTA
425 North LaSalle
Navasota, TX 77868
(409) 825-3624
TDD: (409) 825-1755

ROCKDALE
313 North Main
Rockdale, TX 76567-2999
(512) 446-2543

ROUND ROCK
1011 Gattis School Road
Suites 104 & 110
Round Rock, TX 78664-7048
(512) 244-1592
TDD: (512) 238-0937

SAN MARCOS
1901 Dutton Drive
Suite C
San Marcos, TX 78666-5964
(512) 753-2201 and (512) 753-2246
TDD: (512) 753-2280

SAN SABA
County Annex
412 East Wallace
San Saba, TX 76877-3528
(915) 372-5188

TAYLOR
115 West 6th
Taylor, TX 76574-3551
(512) 352-3611

TAYLOR
301 Highland
Taylor, TX 76574-1848
(512) 352-7661

TEAGUE
1320 US Highway 84 West
Teague, TX 75860-5114
(254) 739-2572

TEMPLE
102 East Central
Temple, TX 76501-4318
(254) 778-6751
TDD: (254) 770-2611

TEMPLE
301 North 3rd
Suite A
Temple, TX 76501-3160
(254) 742-2955
TDD: (254) 742-3843

WACO
801 Austin Avenue
Waco, TX 76701-1935
(254) 775-7656
TDD: (254) 750-9691

WACO
201 West Waco Drive
Waco, TX 76707-3859
(254) 756-6111
TDD: (254) 750-1180

WACO
2010 LaSalle
Waco, TX 76706
(254) 752-4839
TDD: (254) 750-7898

WACO
1711 Herring Avenue
Waco, TX 76708-2933
(254) 756-7418
TDD: (254) 750-1080

REGION VIII:

BANDERA
1106 Pecan Street
PO Box 817
Bandera, TX 78003
(210) 796-3739
Fax: (210) 796-7387
Zip Code: 78003

BOERNE
905 North Main
PO Box 1587
Boerne, TX 78006
(210) 249-3533
Zip Code: 78006

BRACKETVILLE
PO Box 176
Bracketville, TX 78832
(210) 563-2473
Fax: (210) 563-2147
Zip Code: 78832

CAMPWOOD
106 North Nueces
Campwood, TX 78833
(210) 597-2183
Fax: (210) 597-3276
Zip Code: 78833

CARRIZO SPRINGS
2208 North First
Carrizo Springs, TX 78834
(210) 876-2456
Fax: (210) 876-3355
Zip Code: 78834

COTULLA
202 North Stewart
Cotulla, TX 78014
(210) 879-3021
Fax: (210) 879-3780
Zip Code: 78014

CRYSTAL CITY
104 Juan Cornejo Drive
Drawer D
Crystal City, TX 78839
(210) 374-2327
Fax: (210) 374-3769
Zip Code: 78839

CUERO
111 East Alexander
PO Box 620
Cuero, TX 79954-0620
(512) 275-2811
Fax: (512) 275-5737
Zip Code: 77974,79954

DEL RIO
801 Bedell
Del Rio, TX 78840
(210) 772-8566

DEL RIO
712 East Gibbs
Del Rio, TX 78840
(210) 774-3661
Zip Code: 78840

DEL RIO
913 South Main
Del Rio, TX 78840
(210) 774-4363

EAGLE PASS
1593 Loop 3443
Eagle Pass, TX 78853
(210) 773-0350
Fax: (210) 773-8619
Zip Code: 78852, 78853

EAGLE PASS
350 South Adams Street
Eagle Pass, TX 78852
(210) 773-5321

EAGLE PASS
2525 Loop 431
PO Box 921
Eagle Pass, TX 78853-0921
(210) 773-5358

EDNA
609 North Wells
Edna, TX 77957-0815
(512) 782-5227
Fax: (512) 782-2843
Zip Code: 77657

FLORESVILLE
661 10th Street
Floresville, TX 78114-3125
(210) 393-3141
Fax: (210) 393-4077
Zip Code: 78112, 78114

FREDERICKSBURG
1904 North Llano
Fredericksburg, TX 78624
(210) 997-7546
Fax: (210) 997-3495
Zip Code: 78624

GOLIAD
105 South Commercial
PO Box Drawer G
Goliad, TX 79936
(512) 645-3732
Fax: (512) 645-3572
Zip Code: 79936

GONZALES
711 Street Joseph
Gonzales, TX 78629
(210) 673-6511
Zip Code: 78629

GONZALES
1600 Sarah Dewitt Drive
Suite 108
Gonzales, TX 78629
(210) 672-6545
Fax: (210) 672-9247
Zip Code: 78629

HALLETTSVILLE
908 North Glendale
PO Drawer G
Hallettsville, TX 77964
(512) 798-3244
Fax: (512) 798-5047
Zip Code: 77964

HONDO
410 Carter Street
PO Box 220
Hondo, TX 78861
(210) 741-2043
Fax: (210) 426-5533
Zip Code: 78861

JOURDANTON
Highway 97 East
Jourdanton, TX 78026
(210) 769-3515

JOURDANTON
1114 Main
Jourdanton, TX 78026-1699
(210) 769-3507
Fax: (210) 769-2572
Zip Code: 78026

KARNES CITY
417 South Panna Maria
PO Box 489
Karnes City, TX 78118
(210) 780-3961
Fax: (210) 780-2512
Zip Code: 78118

KERRVILLE
819 Water Street
Kerrville, TX
(210) 896-3933
Fax: (210) 896-1039
Zip Code: 78028

NEW BRAUNFELS
143 East Garza
New Braunfels, TX 78130
(210) 625-9111

NEW BRAUNFELS
1607 East Common Street
PO Box 311836
New Braunfels, TX 78131-1836
(210) 625-8023
Fax: (210) 625-6416
Zip Code: 78163, 78131

NIXON
603 East Central Avenue
Nixon, TX 78140-3003
(210) 625-6416
Zip Code: 78140

PEARSALL
1009 North Oak
PO Box 1228
Pearsall, TX 78061-1228
(210) 334-3395
Fax: (210) 334-8653
Zip Code: 78061

PLEASANTON
310 West Oaklawn
Pleasanton, TX 78064
(210) 563-2527
Zip Code: 78064

PORT LAVACA
436 North Highway 35
Port Lavaca, TX 77979-1938
(512) 552-9702
Fax: (512) 552-1667
Zip Code: 77979

PORT LAVACA
815 North Virginia
Port Lavaca, TX 77979
(512) 552-6713

SAN ANTONIO
125 Ascot
San Antonio, TX 78224
(210) 927-6883

SAN ANTONIO
4201 Medical Drive
PO Box 23990
San Antonio, TX 78223-0990
(210) 615-8210

SAN ANTONIO
4023 Pleasanton
PO Box 23990
San Antonio, TX 78223-0990
(210) 927-5454
Zip Code: 78221,78224,78263,78264

SAN ANTONIO
3300 Nacogdoches, Suite 140
PO Box 23990
San Antonio, TX 78223-0990
Zip Code: 78213, 78216, 78217, 78218, 78230, 78231, 78232, 78233, 78239, 78247, 78248, 78258, 78259, 78260, 78261

SAN ANTONIO
2711 Palo Alto
PO Box 23990
San Antonio, TX 78223-0990
(210) 977-9720
Zip Codes: 78211,78241,78242

SAN ANTONIO
111 Dallas
San Antonio, TX 78205
(210) 222-8431

SAN ANTONIO
5800 Culebra
PO Box 23990
San Antonio, TX 78223-0990
(210) 431-0225
Zip Code: 78015, 78023, 78201, 78228, 78229, 78238, 78023, 78201, 78228, 78229, 78238, 78255, 78256, 78257

SAN ANTONIO
527 North Leona
San Antonio, TX 78207
(210) 358-3400

SAN ANTONIO
222 Cypress
PO Box 23990
San Antonio, TX 78223-0990
(210) 227-2761
No Zip-Code Applicable

SAN ANTONIO
1028 South Alamo
San Antonio, TX 78210
(210) 731-1300

SAN ANTONIO
8109 Fredericksburg
San Antonio, TX
(210) 692-5000

SAN ANTONIO
519 East Houston
San Antonio, TX 78205
(210) 704-2041

SAN ANTONIO
6711 South New Braunfels
San Antonio, TX 78223
(210) 532-8811

SAN ANTONIO
7400 Barlite
San Antonio, TX 78224
(210) 921-2000

SAN ANTONIO
7700 Floyd Curl Drive
San Antonio, TX 78229
(210) 692-4000

SAN ANTONIO
1102 Barclay
San Antonio, TX 78207
(210) 434-2647

SAN ANTONIO
2534 Castroville
PO Box 23990
San Antonio, TX 78223-0990
(210) 436-4392
Fax: (210) 431-2368
Zip Code: 78039, 78054, 78227, 78236, 78237, 78240, 78245, 78249,
78250, 78251, 78252, 78253, 78254

SAN ANTONIO
404 Brady
PO Box 23990
San Antonio, TX 78223-0990
(210) 212-6986
Fax: (210) 242-7693
Zip Code: 78207, 78225,78226

SAN ANTONIO
905 & 933 Pleasanton
PO Box 23990
San Antonio, TX 78223-0990
(210) 921-6117
Fax: (210) 977-1260
Zip Code: 78204, 78210,78223,78235

SAN ANTONIO
321 North Center
PO Box 23990
San Antonio, TX 78223-0990
(210) 229-9200
Fax: (210) 270-3395
Zip Code: 78101, 78152, 78202, 78202, 78204, 78205, 78208, 78209, 78212, 78215, 78219, 78220, 78222, 78234, 78244, 78246, 78262

SAN ANTONIO
4502 Medical Drive
San Antonio, TX 78229
(210) 358-4000

SAN ANTONIO
3635 SE Military Drive
PO Box 23990
San Antonio, TX 78223-0990
(210) 333-2001
Fax: (210) 337-3185

SCHERTZ
795 Schertz Parkway
Schertz, TX 78154-2413
(210) 659-5826
Fax: (210) 658-7937
Zip Code: 78233, 78266,78108,78109,78148,78150,78154

SEGUIN
1110 North Camp
Seguin, TX 78155
(210) 379-0342
Fax: (210) 372-2167
Zip Code: 78124, 78155

SOMERSET
19575 K Street
Somerset, TX 78069
(210) 701-3800
Fax: (210) 701-4002
Zip Code: 78002, 78052,78069,78073

UVALDE
2201 East Main
Uvalde, TX 77801
(210) 593-4300
Fax: (210) 278-1583
Zip Code: 78801

UVALDE
1025 Garner Field Road
Uvalde, TX 77801
(210) 278-6251

VICTORIA
2601 North Azalea Street
Victoria, TX 77901
(361) 576-1215
Zip Code: 78901,78902,78903,78904,78905

VICTORIA
2603 Hospital Drive
Victoria, TX 77901
(361) 576-2110

VICTORIA
506 East San Antoniom Street
Victoria, TX 77901
(361) 575-7441

YOAKUM
702 Irvine
PO Box 248
Yoakum, TX 77995-0248
(512) 293-3584
Fax: (512) 564-3856
Zip Code: 77995

YORKTOWN
632 West Main
PO Box 515
Yorktown, TX 78164-0515
(512) 564-3737
Fax: (512) 564-3856
Zip Code: 78164

REGION X:

ALPINE
209 West Holland
PO Box 1015
Alpine, TX 79830
(915) 837-3338
Fax: (915) 837-7840
Zip Code: 79734, 79830,79831,79832,79834,79842,79852

CANDELARIA
Highway 34
Candelaria, TX 79843
(915) 837-3338
Fax: (915) 837-7840

CANUTILLO
6621 Doniphan Drive
PO Box M
Canutillo, TX 79835-5005
(915) 877-3112
Fax: (915) 877-6199
TDD: (915) 877-6154
Zip Code: 79835,79932,88021

CLINT
190 North Clint Road
PO Box 839
Clint, TX 79836-0893
(915) 851-5722
Fax: (915) 851-5756
Zip Code: 79836,79949,79927

DELL CITY
102 South Dodson
Dell City, TX 79837
(915) 283-9005
Fax: (915) 283-9015

EL PASO
5150 El Paso Drive
PO Box 981017
El Paso, TX 79998-1017
(915) 775-4566
Fax: (915) 775-4469
TDD: (915) 775-4593

EL PASO
4800 Alberta
El Paso, TX 79905
(915) 545-6587
Fax: (915) 545-6450
All ZIP codes

EL PASO
7100 Gateway East
El Paso, TX 79915
(915) 774-7490
(800) 458-9858

EL PASO

8061 Alameda Avenue
El Paso, TX 79915-4705
(915) 858-8378
Fax: (915) 859-9862
All ZIP codes

EL PASO

5005 Alameda
El Paso, TX 79998
(915) 775-4591
Fax: (915) 775-4446
TDD: (915) 775-4578

EL PASO

1700 North OR
Suite 785
El Paso, TX 79902
(915) 533-4865
Fax: (915) 521-1768
All ZIP codes

EL PASO

4815 Alameda
El Paso, TX 79998
(915) 521-7948
Fax: (915) 521-7947
All ZIP codes

EL PASO
Eastside Office
11295 Edgemere
PO Box 981017
El Paso, TX 79998-1017
(915) 593-0272
(915) 629-3261
Fax: (915) 629-3296
TDD: (915) 629-3291
Zip Code: 79936,79938

EL PASO
Lomaland Office
1314 Lomaland
PO Box 981017
El Paso, TX 79994-0276
(915) 595-6711
(915) 599-5226
Fax: (915) 599-5250
TDD: (915) 599-5264
Zip Code: 79925,79935

EL PASO
Lower Valley Office
215 Padres Street
PO Box 981017
El Paso, TX 79907-6248
(915) 859-9165
Fax: (915) 858-8396
TDD: (915) 858-8385
Zip Code: 79907

EL PASO
Midtown Office 2300 East Yandell
PO Box 981017
El Paso, TX 79907-6248
(915) 534-7314
Fax: (915) 747-4599
TDD: (915) 747-4509
Zip Code: 79902,79903,79912,79922

EL PASO
Northeast Office 9206 McCombs
PO Box 981017
El Paso, TX 79907-6248
(915) 751-7783
(915) 757-4809
Fax: (915) 757-4895
TDD: (915) 757-4861
Zip Code: 70014,79920,799224,79931,79934

EL PASO
Northland Office 5631 Dyer
Suite 300
El Paso, TX 79907-6248
(915) 564-1010
Fax: (915) 564-6004
TDD: (915) 564-6098
Zip Code: 79904,79930

EL PASO
7904 Alameda
PO Box 981017
El Paso, TX 79907-6248
(915) 858-9699
Fax: (915) 858-7777
TDD: (915) 858-7799

EL PASO
700 South Ochoa
El Paso, TX 79901-2927
(915) 545-7053
Fax: (915) 533-4878
All ZIP codes

EL PASO
10301 Gateway West
El Paso, TX 79937
(915) 595-9684
Fax: (915) 595-9779
All ZIP codes

FABENS
Main Street
PO Box 817
Fabens, TX 79938-0817
(915) 764-3394
Fax: (915) 764-2611
Zip Code: 79838,79839,79853

FORT DAVIS
101 Court Street
Fort Davis, TX 79734
(915) 837-3338
Fax: (915) 837-7840

MARATHON
200 South 6th Street
Marathon, TX 79842
See Alpine: (915) 837-3338
Fax: (915) 837-7840

MARFA
101 North Mesa
PO Box 576
Marfa, TX 79843-0576
(915) 729-4331
Fax: (915) 729-4646
Zip Code: 79843,79854

PRESIDIO
Highway 67 at Louvain
PO Box 938
Presidio, TX 79845-0938
(915) 229-3405
Fax: (915) 229-4061
Zip Code: 79843,79845,79846,79850

REDFORD
Highway 67
Redford, TX 79846
See Presidio: (915) 229-3405
Fax: (915) 729-4646

SIERRA BLANCA
109 Milligan
Sierra Blanca, TX 79851
(915) 283-9005
Fax: (915) 283-9015

TERILINGUA
Highway 170
Terilingua, TX 78752
(915) 371-2233
(915) 837-3338
Fax: (915) 837-5646

VALENTINE
409 Bell Avenue
Valentine, TX 79854
(915) 729-4331
Fax: (915) 729-4646

VAN HORN
700 A. Broadway
PO Box 397
Van Horn, TX 79855-0397
(915) 283-9005
Fax: (915) 283-9015
Zip Code: 79737,79838,79839,79841,79847,79851,79854,79855

Region 11 Office Locations:

ALAMO
1003 East Frontage Road
Expressway 83
Alamo, TX 78516
(956) 787-0026
TDD: (956) 787-2587

ALICE
408 North Airport Road
Alice, TX 78332-4002
(361) 664-7490
TDD: (361) 660-2287

ARANSAS PASS
524 South Commercial
Aransas Pass, TX 78336-1810
(361) 758-7631
TDD: (361) 758-6931

BEEVILLE
1800 South Washington
Suite 1
Beeville, TX 78102
(361) 358-9790
TDD: (361) 358-6648

BENAVIDES CIVIC CENTER
Hwy 59
PO Box 419
Benavides, TX 78341-0419
(361) 256-3352

BROWNSVILLE
3025 Boca Chica
Brownsville, TX 78521
(956) 546-8900
TDD: (956) 982-6750

BROWNSVILLE
1755 West Price Road
Brownsville, TX 78520
(956) 541-0183
TDD: (956) 982-6495

CORPUS CHRISTI
4410 Dillon Lane
Suite 28
Corpus Christi, TX 78415
(361) 857-0878
TDD: (361) 878-7675

CORPUS CHRISTI
5155 Flynn Parkway
PO Box 7622
Corpus Christi, TX 78467-7622
(361) 855-9924
TDD: (361) 878-3365

CORPUS CHRISTI
1233 Agnes
Corpus Christi, TX 78401
(361) 888-7762
TDD: (361) 888-8930

DONNA
202 West Highway 83
Donna, TX 78537-3033
(956) 464-8607
TDD: (956) 464-3279

EDINBURG
300 East Canton
Edinburg, TX 78539-2549
(956) 318-0167
TDD: (956) 316-8689

EDINBURG
815 North Closner
Edinburg, TX 78539-2549
(956) 316-2489
TDD: (956) 316-8416

EDINBURG
2520 South "I" Road
PO Box 960
Edinburg, TX 78540-0960
(956) 383-5344
TDD: (956) 316-8381

EDINBURG
106 South 12th
2nd Floor
Edinburg, TX 78539-3857
(956) 381-1397
TDD: (956) 287-1904

ELSA
South Highway 88
PO Box 1509
Elsa, TX 78543-1509
(956) 262-4701
TDD: (956) 262-6317

FALFURRIAS
1200 East Highway 285
PO Box Drawer S
Falfurrias, TX 78355-0919
(361) 325-5621

FREER
Hunt & Carolyn
PO Box 555
Freer, TX 78357-0555
(361) 394-7378

GEORGE WEST
602 Colorado
PO Drawer BB
George West, TX 78022-0710
(361) 449-1823

HARLINGEN
801 North 13th
Sun Valley Mall, Suite 19
Harlingen, TX 78550-5073
(956) 423-3100
TDD: (956) 412-7650

HARLINGEN
2004 West Jefferson
Suite B
Harlingen, TX 78550-5273
(956) 428-8201

HEBBRONVILLE
1402 West Viggie
Hebbronville, TX 78361
(361) 527-3226

KINGSVILLE
1413 East Corral
PO Box 831
Kingsville, TX 78363-0831
(361) 592-9351
TDD: (361) 592-6831

LA JOYA
1 Block South Highway 83
PO Drawer I
La Joya, TX 78560-0200
(956) 585-4841

LAREDO
4410 Highway 359
Laredo, TX 78043
(956) 791-5203
TDD: (956) 717-5388

LAREDO
3804 Casa Blanca Road
Laredo, TX 78041
(956) 722-0571
TDD: (956) 718-0269

LAREDO
1500 North Arkansas
Laredo, TX 78041-3005
(956) 725-5195
TDD: (956) 764-6295

MATHIS
215 South Highway 359
Mathis, TX 78368-2705
(361) 547-3216

MCALLEN
600 South Bicentennial
McAllen, TX 78501-5275
(956) 630-9441
TDD: (956) 971-1235

MCALLEN
900 East Esperanza
McAllen, TX 78501
(956) 971-9124

MCALLEN
2501 West Pecan
McAllen, TX 78501-7335
(956) 682-9915
TDD: (956) 682-5928

MERCEDES
202 West 2nd Street
Mercedes, TX 78570-2704
(956) 565-2692
TDD: (956) 565-9344

MISSION
102 South Bryan Road
Mission, TX 78572
(956) 580-2531
TDD: (956) 580-6283

MISSION
4015 North Conway
Mission, TX 78572
(956) 585-1579
TDD: (956) 580-6477

PHARR
1503 West Polk
Pharr, TX 78577-9984
(956) 787-3131
TDD: (956) 702-5550

PORT ISABEL
1730 West Highway 100
Port Isabel, TX 78578-0188
(956) 943-5417
TDD: (956) 689-1431

PREMONT
106 North Agnes
PO Box 897
Premont, TX 78375-0897
(361) 348-2234

RAYMONDVILLE
100 North Highway 77
Suite I
Raymondville, TX 78580-2599
(956) 689-6501
TDD: (956) 689-1431

REFUGIO
418 North Alamo
Refugio, TX 78377-2504
(361) 526-4627

RIO GRANDE CITY
400 West Eisenhower
Rio Grande City, TX 78582-2599
(956) 487-2537
TDD: (956) 716-6250

ROBSTOWN
429 East Main
Robstown, TX 78380-2207
(361) 387-8051
TDD: (361) 387-6571

ROCKPORT
2718 Highway 35 North
Rockport, TX 78382-5709
(361) 729-5784

ROMA
Margarita Street & US Highway
PO Box 910
Roma, TX 78584-0619
(956) 849-1075
TDD: (956) 849-9095

SAN BENITO
155 East Highway 77
San Benito, TX 78586-5232
(956) 399-2819
TDD: (956) 361-4295

SAN DIEGO
1102 East Highway 44
Suite A
San Diego, TX 78384
(361) 279-3301
TDD: (361) 279-7968

SAN JUAN
1103 North Raul Longoria
San Juan, TX 78589-0088
(956) 783-1251
TDD: (956) 783-0237

SINTON
1115 East Sinton Street
Drawer A
Sinton, TX 78387-0166
(361) 364-1240
TDD: (361) 364-4926

WESLACO
2411 North Texas Boulevard
Suite A
Weslaco, TX 78596-6623
(956) 968-1871
TDD: (956) 969-9277

WESLACO
1110 South Airport Drive
Weslaco, TX 78596
(956) 969-9115
TDD: (956) 973-1290

ZAPATA
1306 Kennedy
PO Box 476
Zapata, TX 78076-0476
(956) 765-4319
TDD: (956) 765-3262

UTAH DEPARTMENT OF HUMAN SERVICES

BEAR RIVER AREA AGENCY ON AGING
170 North Main
Logan, Utah 84321
Phone (435) 752-7242
Fax: (435) 752-6962
Box Elder County, Cache County, Rich County

WEBER HUMAN SERVICES
2650 Lincoln Avenue
Ogden, Utah 84401-3610
Phone (801) 625-3656
Fax: (801) 625-3847
Weber County, Morgan County

DAVIS COUNTY COUNCIL ON AGING COURTHOUSE ANNEX
28 East State
PO Box 618
Farmington, Utah 84025
Phone (801) 451-3370 or 451-3377
Fax: (801) 451-3434

TOOELE CO DIV. OF AGING & ADULT SERVICES
59 East Vine Street
Tooele, Utah 84074
Phone (435) 882-2870
Fax: (435) 882-6971

MOUNTAINLAND DEPARTMENT OF AGING & ADULT SERVICES
2545 North Canyon Road
Provo, Utah 84604-5906
Phone (801) 377-2262 or
(801) 377-2263
Fax: (801) 377-2317
Summit County, Utah County, Wasatch County

UINTAH BASIN AREA AGENCY ON AGING
855 East 200 North (112-3)
Roosevelt, Utah 84066
Phone (435) 722-4519
Fax: (435) 722-4890
Daggett County, Duchesne County

UINTAH COUNTY AREA AGENCY ON AGING
155 South 100 West
Vernal, Utah 84078
Phone (435) 789-2169
Fax: (435) 789-2171

ADMINISTRATIVE OFFICE
120 N 200 W
PO Box 142700
Salt Lake City, Utah 84114-2700
Phone (801) 538-3910
Fax: (801) 538-3959

SALT LAKE COUNTY
Six-County Area Agency on Aging
250 North Main, Room 5
PO Box 820
Richfield, Utah 84701
Phone (435) 896-9222
Fax: (435) 896-6951
Juab County, Sanpete County, Millard County, Sevier County, Piute County, Wayne County

SOUTHEASTERN UTAH AAA
375 South Carbon Avenue
Technical Assistance Center
PO Drawer 1106
Price, Utah 84501
Phone (435) 637-4268
Fax: (435) 637-5448
Carbon County, Emery County, Grand County

FIVE-COUNTY AREA AGENCY ON AGING
906 North 1400 West
PO Box 1550
Street George, Utah 84770
Phone (435) 673-3548 (Street George)
(435) 586-2975 (Cedar City)
(435) 676-2281 (Panquitch)
Fax: (435) 673-3540
Beaver County, Iron County, Garfield County, Washington County, Kane County

SAN JUAN COUNTY AAA
117 South Main
PO Box 9
Monticello, UT 84535-0009
Phone (435) 587-3225
Fax: (435) 587-2447

VERMONT DEPARTMENT OF SOCIAL WELFARE

ST ALBANS
20 Houghton Street, Room 313
St Albans, VT 05478
802-524-7900
(800) 660-4513

NEWPORT
100 Main Street, Suite 240
Newport, VT 05855
802-334-6504
(800) 775-0526

BURLINGTON
1193 North Avenue, Suite 5
Burlington, VT 05401-2749
(802) 863-7365
(800) 775-0506

RUTLAND
320 ASA Bloomer State Office Bldg
Rutland, VT 05701
(802) 786-5800
(800) 775-0516

HARTFORD
224 Holiday Drive, Suite A
White River Junction, VT 05001-2097
(802) 295-8855
(800) 775-0507

SPRINGFIELD
100 Mineral Street, Suite 201
Springfield, VT 05156
(802) 885-8856
(800) 589-5775

STREET JOHNSBURY
67 Eastern Avenue, Suite 7
Street Johnsbury, VT 05819
(802) 748-5193
(800) 775-0514

BENNINGTON
200 Veterans Memorial Drive
Suite 6
Bennington, VT 05201-1918
(802) 442-8541
(800) 775-0527

BRATTLEBORO
232 Main Street, PO Box 70
Brattleboro, VT 05302
(802) 257-2820
(800) 775-0515

MORRISVILLE
63 Professional Drive
Morrisville, VT 05661
(802) 888-4291
(800) 775-0525

BARRE
255 North Main Street, Suite 5
Barre, VT 05641-4160
(802) 479-1041
(800) 499-0113

MIDDLEBURY
700 Exchange Street, Suite 103
Middlebury, VT 05753-9943
(802) 388-3146
(800) 244-2035

VIRGINIA LOCAL SOCIAL SERVICE AGENCIES

CENTRAL REGIONAL OFFICE
1604 Santa Rosa Road
Wythe Building, Suite 130
Richmond, VA 23229
(804) 662-7653

CAROLINE
PO Box 430
Bowling Green, VA 22427-0430
(804) 633-5071
Fax: (804) 633-5648

WESTMORELAND
Peach Grove Lane
PO Box 302
Montross, VA 22520-0302
(804) 493-9305
Fax: (804) 493-9309

CHARLES CITY
PO Box 98
Charles City, VA 23030-0098
(804) 829-9207
Fax: (804) 829-2430

CHESTERFIELD/COLONIAL HEIGHTS
9501 Lucy Corr Drive
PO Box 430
Chesterfield, VA 23832-0430
(804) 748-1100
Fax: (804) 796-1837

DINWIDDIE
PO Box 107
Dinwiddie, VA 23841
(804) 469-4524
Fax: (804) 469-4506

ESSEX
PO Box 1004
Tappahannock, VA 22560-1004
(804) 443-3561
Fax: (804) 443-8254

FREDERICKSBURG
608 Jackson Street
PO Box 510
Fredericksburg, VA 22404-0510
(540) 372-1032
Fax: (540) 372-1157

GLOUCESTER
PO Box 1390
Gloucester, VA 23061-0186
(804) 693-2671
Fax: (804) 693-5511

GOOCHLAND
Administration Annex Building
PO Box 34
Goochland, VA 23063-0034
(804) 556-5332
Fax: (804) 784-5510
(804) 556-4718

GREENSVILLE/EMPORIA
1748 East Atlantic Street
PO Box 1136
Emporia, VA 23847-1136
(804) 634-6576
Fax: (804) 634-9504

HANOVER
12304 Washington Highway
Ashland, VA 23005
(804) 752-4100
Fax: (800) 770-0837
(804) 752-4110

HENRICO COUNTY
8600 Dixon Powers Drive
PO Box 27032
Richmond, VA 23273
(804) 501-4001
Fax: (804) 501-4006

HOPEWELL
256 East Cawson Street
Hopewell, VA 23860-2804
(804) 541-2330
Fax: (804) 541-2347

KING & QUEEN
PO Box 7
Courthouse Annex
King & Queen Courthouse, VA 23095-9999
(804) 769-5003
(804) 785-5977
Fax: (804) 785-5885

KING GEORGE
PO Box 130
King George, VA 22484-0130
(540) 775-3544
Fax: (540) 775-3098

KING WILLIAM
County Office Building
PO Box 187
King William, VA 23086-0187
(804) 769-4905
Fax: (804) 769-4964

LANCASTER
PO Box 185
Lancaster, VA 22503
(804) 462-5141
Fax: (804) 462-0330

MATHEWS
Route 611
PO Box 925
Mathews, VA 23109-0925
(804) 725-7192
Fax: (804) 725-7086

MIDDLESEX
PO Box 216
Urbanna, VA 23175-0216
(804) 758-2348
Fax: (804) 758-2357

NEW KENT
3610 A North Courthouse Road
PO Box 399
Providence Forge, VA 23140
Fax: (804) 966-1853
(804) 966-9170

NORTH UMBERLAND
HEALTH AND SOCIAL SERVICES BUILDING
PO Box 399
Heathsville, VA 22473-0399
(804) 580-3477
Fax: (804) 580-5815

PETERSBURG
400 Farmer Street
PO Box 2127
Petersburg, VA 23804
(804) 861-4720
(804) 748-8426
Fax: (804) 861-0137

POWHATAN
3908 Old Buckingham Road
PO Box 99
Powhatan, VA 23139-0099
(804) 598-5630
(804) 794-9593
Fax: (804) 598-5614

PRINCE GEORGE
PO Box 68
Prince George, VA 23875-0068
(804) 733-2650
Fax: (804 733-2652

RICHMOND CITY
PO Box 10129
Richmond, VA 23240
(804) 780-7430
Fax: (804) 780-7441

RICHMOND COUNTY
5579 Richmond Road
PO Box 35
Warsaw, VA 22572-0035
(804) 333-4088
Fax: (804) 333-0156

SPOTSYLVANIA
Route #208 Holbert Bldg.
9104 Courthouse Road
PO Box 249
Spotsylvania, VA 22553-0249
(540) 582-7065
Fax: (540) 582-7068

STAFFORD
STAFFORD COUNTY GOVERNMENT CENTER
1300 Courthouse Road
PO Box 7
Stafford, VA 22555-0007
(540) 658-8720
Fax: (540) 658-8798

SURRY
Route 626
PO Box 263
Surry, VA 23883-0263
(757) 294-5240
Fax: (757) 294-5248

SUSSEX
Newsome Building
20103 Princeton Road
PO Box 1336
Sussex, VA 23884-1336
(804) 246-7020
Fax: (804) 246-2504

EASTERN REGIONAL OFFICE
Pembroke IV Office Building
Suite 300
Pembroke Office Park
Virginia Beach, VA 23462
(757) 491-3999
Fax: (757) 552-1832

ACCOMACK
PO Box 299
Onancock, VA 23417-0299
(757) 787-1530
Fax: (757) 787-9303

CHESAPEAKE BUREAU OF SOCIAL SERVICES
100 Outlaw Street, PO Box 15098
Chesapeake, VA 23320
(757) 382-2000
Fax: (757) 543-1644

FRANKLIN DEPARTMENT OF SOCIAL SERVICES
City Hall Annex, 207 West Second Avenue
Franklin, VA 23851
(757) 562-8520
Fax: (757) 562-8515

HAMPTON DEPARTMENT OF SOCIAL SERVICES
1320 LaSalle Avenue
Hampton, VA 23669
(757) 727-1800
Fax: (757) 727-1835

ISLE OF WIGHT DEPARTMENT OF SOCIAL SERVICES
17100 Monument Circle, StEast A
Isle of Wight, VA 23397-0110
(757) 365-0880
Fax: (757) 365-0886

JAMES CITY CO. DEPARTMENT OF SOCIAL SERVICES
5249 Old Towne Road
Williamsburg, VA 23188
(757) 259-3100
Fax: (757) 259-3188

NEWPORT NEWS DEPARTMENT OF SOCIAL SERVICES
Rouse Tower
6060 Jefferson Avenue
Newport News, VA 23605
(757) 926-6300
Fax: (757) 926-6118

NORFOLK DIVISION OF SOCIAL SERVICES
Franklin Building
220 West Brambleton Avenue
Norfolk, VA 23510-1506
(757) 664-6000
Fax: (757) 664-3275

NORTHAMPTON CO DEPARTMENT OF SOCIAL SERVICES
PO Box 568
Eastville, VA 23347-0568
(757) 678-5153
Fax: (757) 678-0475

PORTSMOUTH DEPARTMENT OF SOCIAL SERVICES
1701 High Street
Portsmouth, VA 23704-2417
(757) 398-3600
Fax: (757) 393-5058

SOUTHAMPTON CO DEPARTMENT OF SOCIAL SERVICES
26022 Administration Center Drive
PO Box 550
Courtland, VA 23837-0550
(757) 653-3080
Fax: (757) 653-0357

SUFFOLK DEPARTMENT OF SOCIAL SERVICES
440 Market Street
PO Box 1818
Suffolk, VA 23434-1818
(757) 923-3096
Fax: (757) 923-3047

VIRGINIA BEACH DEPARTMENT OF SOCIAL SERVICES
3432 Virginia Beach Boulevard
Virginia Beach, VA 23452-4420
(757) 437-3200
Fax: (757) 437-3300

WILLIAMSBURG SOCIAL SERVICE BUREAU
401 Lafayette Street
Williamsburg, VA 23185
(757) 220-6161
Fax: (757) 220-6109

YORK-POQUOSON SOCIAL SERVICES
301 Goodwin Neck Road
PO Drawer 917
Yorktown, VA 23692-0917
(757) 890-3930
Fax: (757) 890-3934

NORTHERN REGIONAL OFFICE
320 Hospital Drive, Suite 31
Warrenton, VA 22186
(540) 347-6307

ALBEMARLE COUNTY DEPARTMENT OF SOCIAL SERVICES
401 McIntire Road
Charlottesville, VA 22901
(804) 972-4010

CITY OF WINCHESTER DEPARTMENT OF SOCIAL SERVICES
33 East Boscawen Street
Winchester, VA 22601
(540) 662-3807

CITY OF ALEXANDRIA DEPARTMENT OF SOCIAL SERVICES
2525 Mt Vernon Avenue
Alexandria, VA 22301
(703) 338-0700

ARLINGTON COUNTY DEPARTMENT OF HUMAN SERVICES
180l North George Mason
Post Office Box 7266
Arlington, VA 22207
(703) 228-4994
Fax: (804) 796-1837

BATH COUNTY DEPARTMENT OF SOCIAL SERVICES
Post Office Box 7
Warm Springs, VA 24484
(540) 839-7271

CITY OF CHARLOTTESVILLE DEPARTMENT OF SOCIAL SERVICES
120 7th Street North East
Post Office Box 911
Charlottesville, VA 22902-0911
(804) 970-3400

CLARKE COUNTY DEPARTMENT OF SOCIAL SERVICES
32 East Main Street
Berryville, VA 22611-1338
(540) 955-3700

CULPEPER COUNTY DEPARTMENT OF SOCIAL SERVICES
155 West Davis Street
Culpeper, VA 22701-3046
(540) 727-3436

FAIRFAX COUNTY DEPARTMENT OF FAMILY SERVICES
12011 Government Center Parkway
Suite 200 B-3
Fairfax, VA 22035
(703) 324-7500

FAUQUIER COUNTY DEPARTMENT OF SOCIAL SERVICES
320 Hospital Drive, Suite 11
PO Box 300
Warrenton, VA 20188-0300
(540) 347-2316

FLUVANNA COUNTY DEPARTMENT OF SOCIAL SERVICES
Post Office Box 98
Fork Union, VA 23055
(804) 842-8221

FREDERICK COUNTY DEPARTMENT OF SOCIAL SERVICES
107 North Kent Street, Suite 200
Winchester, VA 22601
(540) 665-5688

GREENE COUNTY DEPARTMENT OF SOCIAL SERVICES
Post Office Box 117
Stanardsville, VA 22973-0117
(804) 985-5246

HARRISONBURG / ROCKINGHAM COUNTY DEPARTMENT OF SOCIAL SERVICES
110 North Mason Street
Post Office Box 809
Harrisonburg, VA 22801
(540) 574-5100

HIGHLAND COUNTY DEPARTMENT OF SOCIAL SERVICES
Courthouse Annex, Post Office Box 247
Monterey, VA 24465-0247
(540) 468-2199

LOUDOUN COUNTY DEPARTMENT OF SOCIAL SERVICES
102 Heritage Way, NE, Suite 200
Leesburg, VA 20176
(703) 777-0353

LOUISA COUNTY DEPARTMENT OF SOCIAL SERVICES
McDonald Street
PO Box 425
Louisa, VA 23093-0425
(540) 967-1320

MADISON COUNTY DEPARTMENT OF SOCIAL SERVICES
101 South Main Street
PO Box 176
Madison, VA 22727-0176
(540) 948-5521

MANASSAS CITY DEPARTMENT OF SOCIAL SERVICES
8955 Center Street
Manassas, VA 20110
(703) 361-8277

MANASSAS PARK DEPARTMENT OF SOCIAL SERVICES
City Hall
1 Park Center Court
Manassas Park, VA 20111
(703) 335-8680

NELSON COUNTY DEPARTMENT OF SOCIAL SERVICES
Court St, Post Office Box 357
Lovingston, VA 22949
(804) 263-8334

ORANGE COUNTY DEPARTMENT OF SOCIAL SERVICES
146 Madison Road, Suite 201
Orange, VA 22960
(540) 672-1155
(804) 748-8426
Fax: (804) 861-0137

PAGE COUNTY DEPARTMENT OF SOCIAL SERVICES
2 Mechanic Street
Luray, VA 22835
(540) 743-6568

PRINCE WILLIAM COUNTY DEPARTMENT OF SOCIAL SERVICES
7987 Ashton Avenue, Suite 200
Manassas, VA 20109
(703) 792-7500

RAPPAHANNOCK COUNTY DEPARTMENT OF SOCIAL SERVICES
PO Box 87
Washington, VA 22747-0087
(540) 675-3313

ROCKBRIDGE / BUENA VISTA / LEXINGTON AREA SOCIAL SERVICES
20 East Preston Street
Lexington, VA 24450
(540) 463-7143

SHENANDOAH COUNTY DEPARTMENT OF SOCIAL SERVICES
236 South Main Street
Post Office Box 192
Woodstock, VA 22664-0192
(540) 459-3736

STAUTON / AUGUSTA COUNTY DEPARTMENT OF SOCIAL SERVICES
4801 Lee Highway
PO Box 7
Verona, VA 24482
(540) 245-5800

WARREN COUNTY DEPARTMENT OF SOCIAL SERVICES
912 Warren Avenue
Post Office Box 506
Front Royal, VA 22630-0506
(540) 635-3430

CITY OF WAYNESBORO DEPARTMENT OF SOCIAL SERVICES
401 Spring Lane
Post Office Box 1028
Waynesboro, VA 22980
(540) 942-6646

PIEDMONT REGIONAL OFFICE
Commonwealth Building, Suite 100
210 Church Avenue, SouthWest
Roanoke, VA 24011
(540) 857-7965
Fax: (540) 857-7364

ALLEGHANY-COVINGTON DEPARTMENT OF SOCIAL SERVICES
110 Rosedale Avenue
Covington, VA 24426-1244
(540) 965-1780
Fax: (540) 965-1606

AMELIA DEPARTMENT OF SOCIAL SERVICES
Court Street
PO Box 136
Amelia, VA 23002-0136
(804) 561-2681
Fax: (540) 561-6040

AMHERST DEPARTMENT OF SOCIAL SERVICES
400 Second Street
PO Box 414
Amherst, VA 24521-0414
(804) 946-9330
Fax: (804) 946-9319

APPOMATTOX DEPARTMENT OF SOCIAL SERVICES
Court Street
PO Box 549
Appomattox, VA 24552-0549
(804) 352-7125
Fax: (804) 352-0064

BEDFORD DEPARTMENT OF SOCIAL SERVICES
Burks-Scott Building
119 East Main Street
Bedford, VA 24523-2095
(540) 586-7750
Fax: (540) 586-7785

BOTETOURT COUNTY DEPARTMENT OF SOCIAL SERVICES
20 South Roanoke Street, Suite 100
PO Box 160
Fincastle, VA 24090-0160
(540) 473-8210
Fax: (540) 473-8325

BRUNSWICK COUNTY DEPARTMENT OF SOCIAL SERVICES
228 North Main Street, Room 301
Lawrenceville, VA 23868-0089
(804) 848-2142
Fax: (804) 848-2828

BUCKINGHAM COUNTY DEPARTMENT OF SOCIAL SERVICES
Route 60
PO Box 170
Buckingham, VA 23921-0170
(804) 969-4246
Fax: (804) 969-1449

CAMPBELL COUNTY DEPARTMENT OF SOCIAL SERVICES
Route 838
PO Box 6
Rustburg, VA 24588-0006
(804) 332-9585
Fax: (804) 332-1707

CHARLOTTE COUNTY DEPARTMENT OF SOCIAL SERVICES
Highway 147
PO Drawer 440
Charlotte Court House, VA 23923-0040
(804) 542-5164
Fax: (804) 542-5248

CLIFTON FORGE DEPARTMENT OF SOCIAL SERVICES
537 Main Street
PO Box 58
Clifton Forge, VA 24422-0058
(540) 863-2525
Fax: (540) 863-2532

CRAIG COUNTY DEPARTMENT OF SOCIAL SERVICES
Main and Court Streets
PO Box 330
New Castle, VA 24127-0330
(540) 864-5117
Fax: (540) 864-6662

CUMBERLAND COUNTY DEPARTMENT OF SOCIAL SERVICES
Route 60
PO Box 33
Cumberland, VA 23040-9803
(540) 492-4915
Fax: (804) 492-9346

DANVILLE DIVISION OF SOCIAL SERVICES
510 Patton Street
PO Box 3300
Danville, VA 24543
(804) 799-6543
Fax: (804) 797-8818

FRANKLIN COUNTY DEPARTMENT OF SOCIAL SERVICES
11161 Virgil H. Goode Highway
Rocky Mount, VA 24151
(540) 483-9247
Fax: (540) 483-1933

HALIFAX COUNTY DEPARTMENT OF SOCIAL SERVICES
Mary Bethune Complex-Cowford Building
PO Box 1189
Halifax, VA 24558-0666
(804) 476-6594
Fax: (804) 476-5258

HENRY COUNTY/MARTINSVILLE DEPARTMENT OF SOCIAL SERVICES
20 East Church Street
PO Drawer 832
Martinsville, VA 24114
(540) 656-4300
Fax: (540) 656-4303

LUNENBURG COUNTY DEPARTMENT OF SOCIAL SERVICES
Courthouse Square
Lunenburg, VA 23952-9999
(804) 696-2134
Fax: (804) 696-2534

LYNCHBURG DIVISION OF SOCIAL SERVICES
2210 Langhorne Road
Lynchburg, VA 24501
(804) 847-1531
Fax: (804) 847-1353

MECKLENBURG COUNTY DEPARTMENT OF SOCIAL SERVICES
132-133 Washington Street
PO Box 400
Boydton, VA 23917-0400
(804) 738-6138
Fax: (804) 738-6191, Ext 298

NOTTOWAY COUNTY DEPARTMENT OF SOCIAL SERVICES
State Route 625
PO Box 26
Nottoway, VA 23955-0026
(804) 645-8494
Fax: (804) 645-8667

PATRICK COUNTY DEPARTMENT OF SOCIAL SERVICES
106 Rucker Street, Suite 128
Stuart, VA 24171-0498
(540) 694-3328
Fax: (540) 694-4249

PITTSYLVANIA COUNTY DEPARTMENT OF SOCIAL SERVICES
18 Depot Street
PO Drawer E
Chatham, VA 24531-0940
(804) 432-7281
Fax: (804) 432-0923

PRINCE EDWARD DEPARTMENT OF SOCIAL SERVICES
111 South Street
PO Drawer 628
Farmville, VA 23901-0628
(804) 392-3113
Fax: (804) 392-8453

ROANOKE CITY DEPARTMENT OF SOCIAL SERVICES
215 West Church Avenue, Room 307
Roanoke, VA 24011
(540) 853-2894
Fax: (540) 853-2027

ROANOKE COUNTY DEPARTMENT OF SOCIAL SERVICES
220 East Main Street
PO Box 1127
Salem, VA 24153-1127
(540) 387-6087
Fax: (540) 387-6210

WESTERN REGIONAL OFFICE
19 Patton Street
Abingdon, VA 24210
(540) 676-5490
Fax: (540)-676-5621

BLAND COUNTY DEPARTMENT OF SOCIAL SERVICES
Old Bank Building
Bland, VA 24315-0055
(540) 688-4111
Fax: (540) 688-4114

WYTHE COUNTY DEPARTMENT OF SOCIAL SERVICES
275 South 4th Street
Wytheville, VA 24383-2597
(540) 228-5493 and (540) 228-5912
Fax: (540) 228-9272

BRISTOL CITY DEPARTMENT OF SOCIAL SERVICES
621 Washington Street
Bristol, VA 24201-4644
(540) 645-7450
Fax: (540) 645-7475

BUCHANAN COUNTY DEPARTMENT OF SOCIAL SERVICES
Route 5, Box 108E
Grundy, VA 24614-0674
(540) 935-8106
Fax: (540) 935-5412

CARROLL COUNTY DEPARTMENT OF SOCIAL SERVICES
605-8 Pine Street
Hillsville, VA 24343
(540) 728-9186
Fax: (540) 728-9987

DICKENSON COUNTY DEPARTMENT OF SOCIAL SERVICES
Brush Creek Road
PO Box 417
Clintwood, VA 24228-0417
(540) 926-1661 and (540) 926-1664
Fax: (540) 926-8144

FLOYD COUNTY DEPARTMENT OF SOCIAL SERVICES
Courthouse Building
PO Box 314
Floyd, VA 24091-0314
(540) 745-9316

GALAX CITY DEPARTMENT OF SOCIAL SERVICES
PO Box 166, 105 E Center St
Galax, VA 24333-0166
(540) 236-8111
Fax: (540) 236-9313

GILES COUNTY DEPARTMENT OF SOCIAL SERVICES
Highway 460
PO Box 529
Pembroke, VA 24136
(540) 626-7291
Fax: (540) 626-7911

GRAYSON COUNTY DEPARTMENT OF SOCIAL SERVICES
PO Box 434, 129 Davis Street
Independence, VA 24348-0434
(540) 773-2452
Fax: (540) 773-2361

LEE COUNTY DEPARTMENT OF SOCIAL SERVICES
PO Box 348, Main Street
Jonesville, VA 24263-0346
(540) 346-1010
Fax: (540) 346-2217

MONTGOMERY COUNTY DEPARTMENT OF SOCIAL SERVICES
210 South Pepper Street
PO Box 789
Christiansburg, VA 24073
(540) 382-6990
Fax: (540) 382-6945

NORTON CITY DEPARTMENT OF SOCIAL SERVICES
644 Park Avenue
PO Box 378
Norton, VA 24273-0378
(540) 679-4393 and (540) 679-2701
Fax: (540)-679-0607

PULASKI COUNTY DEPARTMENT OF SOCIAL SERVICES
143 Third Street, NW
PO Box 110
Pulaski, VA 24301-0110
(540) 980-7995

RADFORD CITY DEPARTMENT OF SOCIAL SERVICES
208 Third Avenue
Radford, VA 24141-4706
(540) 731-3663
Fax: (540) 731-5000

RUSSELL COUNTY DEPARTMENT OF SOCIAL SERVICES
155 Combs Street
PO Box 1207
Lebanon, VA 24266-1207
(540) 889-2679 and (540) 889-3031
Fax: (540) 889-2662

SCOTT COUNTY DEPARTMENT OF SOCIAL SERVICES
PO Box 637
Gate City, VA 24251-0637
(540) 386-3631/6031
Fax: (540) 386-4001

SMYTH COUNTY DEPARTMENT OF SOCIAL SERVICES
121 Bagley Circle, Suite 200
Marion, VA 24354
(540) 783-8148
Fax: (540) 783-6327

TAZWELL COUNTY DEPARTMENT OF SOCIAL SERVICES
PO Box 149
Tazwell, VA 24651
(540) 988-2521
Fax: (540) 988-2765

WASHINGTON COUNTY DEPARTMENT OF SOCIAL SERVICES
15068 Lee Highway, Suite 100
Bristol, VA 24201
(540) 623-2661
Fax: (540) 645-5055

WISE COUNTY DEPARTMENT OF SOCIAL SERVICES
Coeburn Mountain Road
PO Box 888
Wise, VA 24293-0888
(540) 329-8056 and (540) 329-8057
Fax: (540)-328-8632

VIRGIN ISLANDS (US)
No information available, other than the following address/phone numbers available from the Health Care Financing Administration Medicaid Officials Webpage. Please contact for details on Medicaid Eligibility.

VIRGIN ISLANDS DEPARTMENT OF HUMAN SERVICES
Government of the Virgin Islands
Knud Hansen Complex, Bldg A
1303 Hospital Ground
Saint Thomas, VI 00802
(304) 774-0930
Fax: (304) 774-3466

VIRGIN ISLANDS DEPARTMENT OF HEALTH
Government of the Virgin Islands
48 Sugar Estate
Saint Thomas, VI 00802

BUREAU OF HEALTH INSURANCE AND MEDICAL ASSISTANCE
Priscilla Berry, Director
(340) 774-4624

WASHINGTON

HEADQUARTERS
Community Services Division
PO Box 45440
Olympia, WA 98504-5440
Telephone: (360) 413-3370
Fax: (360) 413-3491

REGION 1

REGIONAL HEADQUARTERS
1011 East Second, Suite 8
Spokane, WA 99202
Telephone: (509) 533-2400
Fax: (509) 533-2517
Counties served: Adams, Asotin, Chelan, Douglas, Ferry, Garfield, Grant, Lincoln, Okanogan, Pend Oreille, Spokane, Stevens, Whitman

ADAMS COUNTY
Grant/Adams CSO (Moses Lake)
1620 South Pioneer Way
Moses Lake, WA 98837
Telephone: (509) 764-5600
Fax: (509) 764-5747

OTHELLO BRANCH OFFICE
1025 First Street
PO Box 711
Othello, WA 99344
Telephone: (509) 488-9673
Fax: (509) 488-5068

ASOTIN COUNTY
Clarkston CSO
525 Fifth Street
Clarkston, WA 99403
Telephone: (509) 758-5537
Fax: (509) 758-4582

CHELAN COUNTY
Wenatchee CSO
805 South Mission
PO Box 3088
Wenatchee, WA 98807
Telephone: (509) 662-0511, 662-0541
Fax: (509) 664-6340

DOUGLAS COUNTY
Wenatchee CSO
805 South Mission
PO Box 3088
Wenatchee, WA 98807
Telephone: (509) 662-0511
Fax: (509) 664-6340

FERRY COUNTY
Tri-County CSO
1100 South Main
Colville, WA 99114
Telephone: (509) 685-5600
Fax: (509) 685-5606

Republic Outstation
147 North Clark Avenue
PO Box 1037
Republic, WA 99166
Telephone: (509) 775-3155
Fax: (509) 775-2401

GARFIELD COUNTY
Clarkston CSO
525 Fifth Street
Clarkston, WA 99403
Telephone: (509) 758-5537
Fax: (509) 758-4582

GRANT COUNTY
Grant/Adams CSO (Moses Lake)
1620 South Pioneer Way
Moses Lake, WA 98837
Telephone: (509) 764-5600
Fax: (509) 764-5747

LINCOLN COUNTY
Davenport Branch Office
506 Eighth Street
PO Box 640
Davenport, WA 99122
Telephone: (509) 725-5501, 456-6116
Fax: (509) 725-2056

OKANOGAN COUNTY
Okanogan CSO
130 South Main
PO Box 3729
Omak, WA 98841
Telephone: (509) 826-7200
Fax: (509) 826-7293

PEND OREILLE COUNTY
Tri-County CSO
1100 South Main
Colville, WA 99114
Telephone: (509) 685-5600
Fax: (509) 685-5606

NEWPORT BRANCH OFFICE
1600 West First Street
PO Box 570
Newport, WA 99156-0570
Telephone: (509) 447-3192
Fax: (509) 447-4732

SPOKANE COUNTY
Spokane Central Support CSO
1313 North Maple Street
Spokane, WA 99201-1935
Telephone: (509) 456-4404
Fax: (509) 456-2461

COLF BRANCH OFFICE
418 South Main, Suite 1
Colf, WA 99111
Telephone: (509) 397-4326
Fax: (509) 397-3498

SPOKANE EAST CSO
121 South Arthur
PO Box 2640
Spokane, WA 99202
Telephone: (509) 533-2326
Fax: (509) 533-2343

SPOKANE NORTH CSO
1925 East Francis
Spokane, WA 99207
Telephone: (509) 483-5696
Fax: (509) 483-5716

SPOKANE SOUTHWEST CSO
1313 North Maple
Spokane, WA 99201-2749
Telephone: (509) 458-2191
Fax: (509) 456-3093

DAVEN PORT BRANCH OFFICE
506 Eighth Street
PO Box 640
Davenport, WA 99122
Telephone: (509) 725-5501
Fax: (509) 725-2056

STEVENS COUNTY
Tri-County CSO
1100 South Main
Colville, WA 99114
Telephone: (509) 685-5600
Fax: (509) 685-5606

WHITMAN COUNTY
Clarkston CSO
525 Fifth Street
Clarkston, WA 99403
Telephone: (509) 758-5537
Fax: (509) 758-4582

REGION 2

REGIONAL HEADQUARTERS
1002 North 16th Avenue
PO Box 9428
Yakima, WA 98909
Telephone: (509) 225-7900
Fax: (509) 575-2903
Counties served: Benton, Columbia, Franklin, Kittitas, Walla Walla, Yakima

BENTON COUNTY
Grandview CSO
1313 West Wine Country Road
PO Box 70
Grandview, WA 98930-0070
Telephone: (509) 882-9300
Fax: (509) 882-4589

KENNEWICK CSO
1120 North Edison Avenue
PO Box 6330
Kennewick, WA 99336
Telephone: (509) 735-7119
Fax: (509) 736-2857

COLUMBIA COUNTY
Walla Walla CSO
416 East Main
PO Box 517
Walla Walla, WA 99362
Telephone: (509) 529-0406
Fax: (509) 522-4330

FRANKLIN COUNTY
Pasco CSO
800 West Court
PO Box 931
Pasco, WA 99301
Telephone: (509) 545-1400
Fax: (509) 546-2414

KITTITAS COUNTY
Yakima/Kittitas CSO
1002 North 16th Avenue
PO Box 12500
Yakima, WA 98909
Telephone: (509) 225-6210
Fax: (509) 575-2088

ELLENSBURG BRANCH OFFICE
521 Mountain View
PO Box 366
Ellensburg, WA 98926
Telephone: (509) 962-7710
Fax: (509) 962-7736

WALLA WALLA COUNTY
Walla Walla CSO
416 East Main
PO Box 517
Walla Walla, WA 99362
Telephone: (509) 529-0406
Fax: (509) 522-4330

YAKIMA COUNTY
Grandview CSO
1313 West Wine Country Road
PO Box 70
Grandview, WA 98930-0070
Telephone: (509) 882-9300
Fax: (509) 882-4589

SUNNYSIDE CSO
810 East Custer Avenue
PO Box 818
Sunnyside, WA 98944
Telephone: (509) 837-3531
Fax: (509) 839-7224

TOPPENISH CSO
306 Bolin Drive
PO Box 470
Toppenish, WA 98948
Telephone: (509) 865-2805
Fax: (509) 865-1133

WAPATO CSO
102 North Wapato Avenue
PO Box 66
Wapato, WA 98951
Telephone: (509) 877-8122
Fax: (509) 877-8149

YAKIMA CSO
1002 North 16th Avenue
PO Box 12500
Yakima, WA 98909
Telephone: (509) 225-6100
Fax: (509) 454-4332

YAKIMA/KITTITAS CSO
1002 North 16th Avenue
PO Box 12500
Yakima, WA 98909
Telephone: (509) 225-6210
Fax: (509) 575-2088

REGION 3

REGIONAL HEADQUARTERS
840 North Broadway
Suite 300
Everett, WA 98201-1295
Telephone: (425) 339-3995
Fax: (425) 339-3888
Counties served: Island, San Juan, Skagit, Snohomish, Whatcom

ISLAND COUNTY
Oak Harbor CSO
656 SE Bayshore Drive, #1
Oak Harbor, WA 98277-0909
Telephone: (360) 240-4700
Fax: (360) 679-3524

SAN JUAN COUNTY
Friday Harbor Outstation
55 Second Street, Suite 101
PO Box 1215
Friday Harbor, WA 98250
Telephone: (360) 378-4196
Fax: (360) 378-4098

SKAGIT COUNTY
Mount Vernon CSO
900 East College Way, Suite 100
Mount Vernon, WA 98273-5682
Telephone: (360) 416-7444
Fax: (360) 416-7279

SNOHOMISH COUNTY
Alderwood CSO
19000 33rd Avenue West
PO Box 97012
Lynnwood, WA 98046-9712
Telephone: (425) 673-3000
Fax: (425) 672-2295

EVERETT CSO
840 North Broadway
Suite 200
Everett, WA 98201-1297
Telephone: (425) 339-4000
Fax: (425) 339-4890

SKYKOMISH VALLEY CSO
19705 SR 2
PO Box 7000
Monroe, WA 98272
Telephone: (360) 794-1350
Fax: (360) 794-1360

SMOKEY POINT CSO
3704 172nd Street NE, Suite P
PO Box 3099
Arlington, WA 98223-3099
Telephone: (360) 658-2200
Fax: (360) 658-2294

WHATCOM COUNTY
Bellingham CSO
4101 Meridian Street
PO Box 9706
Bellingham, WA 98227-9706
Telephone: (360) 714-4000
Fax: (360) 714-4066

REGION 4

REGIONAL HEADQUARTERS
400 Mercer Street
Suite 600
Seattle, WA 98109-4641
Telephone: (206) 298-4400
Fax: (206) 298-4601
Counties served: King

KING COUNTY
Holgate-Renton CSO
Physical:
500 SW 7th St, Suite B
Renton, WA 98055
Mailing:
PO Box 94107
Seattle, WA 98124-6407
Telephone: (425) 793-5700
Fax: (425) 277-7297

BELLTOWN CSO
2106 Second Avenue
Seattle, WA 98121-2298
Telephone: (206) 956-3353
Fax: (206) 956-3360

BURIEN CSO
15811 Ambaum Boulevard SouthWest
Seattle, WA 98166-3090
Telephone: (206) 439-5300
Fax: (206) 439-5324

WEST SEATTLE CSO
4045 Delridge Way SW, Suite #300
Seattle, WA 98106
Telephone: (206) 933-3300
Fax: (206) 933-3315

CAPITOL HILL CSO
1700 East Cherry
Seattle, WA 98122-4694
Telephone: (206) 568-5510
Fax: (206) 720-3189

KING EASTSIDE CSO
14360 SE Eastgate Way
Bellevue, WA 98008-0429
Telephone: (206) 649-4000
Fax: (206) 649-4058

BALLARD CSO
907 North West Ballard Way
Seattle, WA 98107-4683
Telephone: (206) 789-5200
Fax: (206) 706-4252

LAKE CITY CSO
11536 Lake City Way North East
Seattle, WA 98125-5395
Telephone: (206) 368-7200
Fax: (206) 368-7189

KING SOUTH CSO
25316 74th Avenue South
PO Box 848
Kent, WA 98032-0848
Telephone: (253) 872-2145
Fax: (253) 872-2735

FEDERAL WAY CSO
1617 South 324th
PO Box 4629
Federal Way, WA 98063-4629
Telephone: (253) 661-4932
Fax: (253) 661-4904

RAINIER CSO
3600 South Graham
Seattle, WA 98118-3034
Telephone: (206) 760-2000
Fax: (206) 760-2345

REGION 5

REGIONAL HEADQUARTERS
2121 South State, 1st Floor West
Tacoma, WA 98405-2844
Telephone: (253) 593-2300
Fax: (253) 593-2233
Counties served: Kitsap, Pierce

KITSAP COUNTY
Bremerton CSO
4710 Auto Center Blvd.
Bremerton, WA 98312-3300
Telephone: (360) 478-4995
Fax: (360) 478-6960

PIERCE COUNTY

PIERCE NORTH CSO
1949 South State Street, 2nd Floor
Tacoma, WA 98405-9945
Telephone: (253) 593-2950
Fax: (253) 597-4319

PIERCE SOUTH CSO
1301 East 72nd
Tacoma, WA 98404-3348
Telephone: (253) 471-4400
Fax: (253) 471-4411

PIERCE WEST CSO
1949 South State Street, 1st Floor
Tacoma, WA 98405-9943
Telephone: (253) 593-2760
Fax: (253) 593-2313

PUYALLUP VALLEY CSO
1004 East Main
Puyallup, WA 98372-9987
Telephone: (253) 840-4600
Fax: (253) 840-4715

REGION 6

REGIONAL HEADQUARTERS
112 Henry Street NE, 3rd Floor
PO Box 45450
Olympia, WA 98504-5450
Telephone: (360) 753-4148
Fax: (360) 586-6367
Counties served: Clallam, Clark, Cowlitz, Grays Harbor, Jefferson, Klickitat, Lewis, Mason, Pacific, Skamania, Thurston, Wahkiakum

CLALLAM COUNTY
Port Angeles CSO
1020 East Front Street
PO Box 2259
Port Angeles, WA 98362-0292
Telephone: (360) 452-3381
Fax: (360) 417-1461

NEAH BAY OUTSTATION
Bayview Avenue, Community Building
PO Box 153
Neah Bay, WA 98357
Telephone: (360) 645-2569
Fax: (360) 645-2452

FORKS BRANCH OFFICE
421 Fifth Avenue South West
Forks, WA 98331
Telephone: (360) 374-2257
Fax: (360) 374-5464

CLARK COUNTY
Orchards CSO
11900 North East 95th Street, Building 4
PO Box 4485
Vancouver, WA 98662
Telephone: (360) 260-6400
Fax: (360) 260-6423

VANCOUVER CSO
907 Harney Street
PO Box 751
Vancouver, WA 98666
Telephone: (360) 993-7700
Fax: (360) 696-6406

COWLITZ COUNTY

KELSO CSO
711 Vine
PO Box 330
Kelso, WA 98626-0026
Telephone: (360) 577-2001
Fax: (360) 577-2296

GRAYS HARBOR COUNTY
Aberdeen CSO
415 West Wishkah
PO Box 189
Aberdeen, WA 98520
Telephone: (360) 537-2600
Fax: (360) 533-9445

ELMA BRANCH OFFICE
575 East Main, Suite A
PO Box 799
Elma, WA 98541
Telephone: (360) 482-8900
Fax: (360) 482-2850

JEFFERSON COUNTY
Port Townsend Branch Office
623 Sheridan
PO Box 554
Port Townsend, WA 98368
Telephone: (360) 379-4300
Fax: (360) 379-5017

KLICKITAT COUNTY
Goldendale Branch Office
808 South Columbus
PO Box 85
Goldendale, WA 98620
Telephone: (509) 773-5835
Fax: (509) 773-4282

WHITE SALMON BRANCH OFFICE
221 North Main
PO Box 129
White Salmon, WA 98672
Telephone: (509) 493-1012
Fax: (509) 493-1882

LEWIS COUNTY
Chehalis CSO
2025 North East Kresky Road
PO Box 359
Chehalis, WA 98532
Telephone: (360) 740-3800
Fax: (360) 748-2286

MASON COUNTY

SHELTON CSO
2505 Olympic Highway N, Suite 440
PO Box 1127
Shelton, WA 98584-0937
Telephone: (360) 432-2000
Fax: (360) 427-2010

PACIFIC COUNTY
South Bend Branch Office
725 West Robert Bush Drive
PO Box 87
South Bend, WA 98586
Telephone: (360) 875-6501
Fax: (360) 875-0590

LONG BEACH BRANCH OFFICE
603 South OR
PO Box 429
Long Beach, WA 98631
Telephone: (360) 642-3791
Fax: (360) 642-6229

SKAMANIA COUNTY

STEVENSON BRANCH OFFICE
266 SW Second Street
PO Box 817
Stevenson, WA 98648
Telephone: (509) 427-5611
Fax: (509) 427-4604

THURSTON COUNTY

OLYMPIA CSO
5000 Capitol Boulevard
PO Box 1908
Olympia, WA 98507-1908
Telephone: (360) 753-5983
Fax: (360) 586-6787

WAHKIAKUM COUNTY

KELSO CSO
711 Vine
PO Box 330
Kelso, WA 98626-0026
Telephone: (360) 577-2001
Fax: (360) 577-2296

WEST VIRGINIA DEPARTMENT OF HEALTH AND HUMAN RESOURCES

REGIONAL/COUNTY OFFICES

REGION I

Counties: Brooke, Calhoun, Doddridge, Gilmer, Hancock, Harrison, Marion, Marshall, Mongalia,Ohio, Pleasants, Ritch, Tyler, Wetzel, Wirt, Wood
107-109 Adams Street
Fairmont, WV 26555
(304) 363-3261
Fax: (304) 367-2729

County Offices for Region 1:

CALHOUN/GILMER/WIRT

404 Main Street
Grantsville, WV 26147
(304) 354-6118
Fax: (304) 354-7076

HANCOCK/BROOKE

213 Three Springs Drive
Weirton, WV 26062
(304) 723-5900
Fax: (304) 723-4133

HARRISON/DODDRIDGE

633 West Pike Street
Clarksburg, WV 26302
(304) 627-2295
Fax: (304) 627-2171

MARION/MONONGALIA
107-109 Adams Street
Fairmont, WV 26555
(304) 363-3261
Fax: (304) 363-5541

MARSHALL
400 Teletech Drive, Suite 2
Moundsville, WV 26041
(304) 843-4120
Fax: (304) 843-4127

OHIO
407 Main Street
Wheeling, WV 26003
(304) 232-4411
Fax: (304) 232-4773

RITCHIE/PLEASANTS
220 West Main Street
Harrisville, WV 26362
(304) 455-0920
Fax: (304) 643-4098

WETZEL/TYLER
331 Main Street
New Martinsville, WV 26155
(304) 455-0920
Fax: (304) 455—029

WOOD
400 Fifth Street
Parkersburg, WV 26102
(304) 485-8461
Fax: (304) 485-1149

REGION II

Counties: Boone, Cabell, Clay, Jackson, Kanawha, Lincoln, Logan, Mason, Mingo, Putnam, Roane, Wayne 4190 West Washington Street
Charleston, WV 25313
(304) 558-9123
Fax: (304) 558-1802

COUNTY OFFICES FOR REGION II

BOONE
Route 3 East
Danville, WV 25053
(304) 369-7802
Fax: (304) 369-7816

CABELL
3135-16th Street
Huntington, WV 25701
(304) 528-5800
Fax: (304) 528-5523

CLAY
Route 4, Box 36A
Clay, WV 25043
(304) 587-4268
Fax: (304) 587-2567

JACKSON/ROANE
2 Academy Drive
Ripley, WV 25271
(304) 372-7885
Fax: (304) 372-7888

KANAWHA
4190 West Washington Street
Charleston, WV 25313
(304) 558-4098
Fax: (304) 558-0851

LINCOLN
8209 Court Avenue
Hamlin, WV 25523
(304) 824-5811
Fax: (304) 824-7811

LOGAN
197 Dingess Street
Logan, WV 25601
(304) 792-7095
Fax: (304) 792-7003

MASON
710 Viand Street
Point Pleasant, WV 25550
(304) 675-0880
Fax: (304) 675-0883

MINGO
PO Box 1820
Williamson, WV 25661
(304) 235-3400
Fax: (304) 235-6020

PUTNAM
PO Box 560
Teays, WV 25569
(304) 757-7843
Fax: (304) 757-8799

WAYNE
PO Box 100
Wayne, WV 25570
(304) 272-6311
Fax: (304) 272-5183

REGION III
Counties: Barbour, Berkeley, Grant, Hampshire, Hardy, Jefferson, Lewis, Mineral, Morgan, Pendleton, Preston, Randolph, Taylor, Tucker, Upshur 15 Grant Street, Suite 1 Petersburg, WV 25402
(304) 257-4211
Fax: (304) 257-1569

County Offices for Region III:

BERKELEY/JEFFERSON/MORGAN
1700 Mid-Atlantic Park
Martinsburg, WV 25402
(304) 267-0100
Fax: (304) 267-0123

HAMPSHIRE/MINERAL
132 West Sioux Lane
Romney, WV 26757
(304) 822-3841
Fax: (304) 822-3846

HARDY/GRANT/PENDLETON
112 Bean's Lane
Moorefield, WV 26836
(304) 538-2391
Fax: (304) 538-2476

LEWIS/UPSHUR
33 East and Smith Run Road
Weston, WV 26452
(304) 269-0532
Fax: (304) 269-0544

RANDOLPH/TUCKER
227 Third Street
Elkins, WV 26241
(304) 637-0333
Fax: (304) 637-0341

TAYLOR/PRESTON/BARBOUR
5 Harmoon Center
Grafton, WV 26354
(304) 265-6103
Fax: (304) 265-6107

REGION IV
Counties: Braxton, Fayette, Greenbrier, McDowell, Mercer, Monroe, Nicholas, Pocahontas, Raleigh, Summers, Webster, Wyoming
Building 6, Room 749
State Capitol Complex
Charleston, WV 25305
(304) 558-0982
Fax: (304) 558-5039

COUNTY OFFICES FOR REGION IV:

BRAXTON
1920 Sutton Lane
Sutton, WV 26601
(304) 765-7344
Fax: (304) 765-3694

FAYETTE
211 West Maple Avenue
Fayetteville, WV 25840
(304) 574-0143
Fax: (304) 574-4129

GREENBRIER/MONROE/POCAHONTAS
150 Maplewood Avenue
Lewisburg, WV 24901
(304) 647-7476
Fax: (304) 647-7486

MCDOWELL
840 Virginia Avenue
Welch, WV 24801
(304) 436-8302
Fax: (304) 436-3248

MERCER
1010 Mercer Street
Princeton, WV 244740
(304) 425-8738
Fax: (304) 487-3589

NICHOLAS
1073 Arbuckle Road
Summersville, WV 26651
(304) 872-0805
Fax: (304) 872-0832

RALEIGH
407 Neville Street
Beckley, WV 25801
(304) 256-6930
Fax: (304) 256-6932

SUMMERS
320 Summers Street, Suite A
Hinton, WV 25951
(304) 466-2807
Fax: (304) 466-2814

WEBSTER
110 North Main Street, Suite 201
Webster Springs, WV 26288
(304) 847-2861
Fax: (304) 847-7244

WYOMING
Box 300
Pineville, WV 24874
(304) 732-6900
Fax: (304) 732-8223

WISCONSIN MEDICAID DEPARTMENTS

ADAMS
(608) 339-3356
(608) 339-4253
Fax: (608) 339-4457
108 East North Street
Post Office Box 500
Friendship, WI 53934-0500

ASHLAND
(715) 682-7004
Fax: (715) 682-7924
301 Ellis Avenue
Ashland, WI 54806

BARRON
(715) 537-5691
Fax: (715) 537-6363
(Barron County DSS)
Courthouse, Room 338
330 East LaSalle Avenue
Barron, WI 54812

BAYFIELD
715) 373-6144
Fax: (715) 373-6130
(Bayfield DHS)
Post Office Box 100
Washburn, WI 54891-0100

BROWN
(920) 448-6460
Fax: (920) 448-6166
Brown County HSD
325 North Rooselvelt Street
Green Bay, WI 54301

BUFFALO
(608) 685-4412
Fax: (608) 685-3342
Buffalo County HS
407 South 2nd Street
Post Office Box 517
Alma, WI 54610-0517

BURNETT
(715) 349-2131
Fax: (715) 349-2145
Burnett County SS
7410 County Road K, #130
Siren, WI 54872

CALUMET COUNTY
(920) 849-1400
Fax: (920) 849-1468
Calumet County HS
206 Court Street
Chilton, WI 53014-1198

CHIPPEWA COUNTY

(715) 726-7840
Fax: (715) 726-7833
Chippewa County HS
711 North Bridge Street, Room 119
Chippewa Falls, WI 54729-1877

CLARK COUNTY

(715) 743-5233
Fax: (715) 743-5242
Clark County SS
517 Court Street
Neillsville, WI 54456

COLUMBIA COUNTY

(608) 742-9227
Fax: (608) 742-9700
Columbia County H&HS
711 East Cook Street
PO Box 136
Portage, WI 53901

CRAWFORD COUNTY

(608) 326-0248
Fax: (608) 326-4395
Crawford County HS
111 West Dunn Street
Prairie du Chien, WI 53821

DANE COUNTY

(608) 242-7441
Fax: (608) 242-7410
Dane County HS
Dane County Connections
1819 Aberg Avenue
Madison, WI 53704

DODGE COUNTY

(920) 386-3750
Fax: (920) 386-3533
Dodge County HS
143 East Center Street
Juneau, WI 53039

DOOR COUNTY

(920) 746-2300
Fax: (920) 746-2355
Door County SS
421 Nebraska Street
Post Office Box 670
Sturgeon Bay, WI 54235-0670

DOUGLAS COUNTY

(715) 395-1241
Fax: (715) 395-1257
Douglas County HS
Courthouse Annex
1313 Belknap Street
Superior, WI 54880

DUNN COUNTY
(715) 232-1116
Fax: (715) 232-5987
Dunn County HS
808 Main Street
Post Office Box 470
Menomonie, WI 54751

EAU CLAIRE COUNTY
(715) 831-5700
Fax: (715) 831-5658
Eau Claire County HS
721 Oxford Avenue
Post Office Box 840
Eau Claire, WI 54702-0840

FLORENCE COUNTY
(715) 528-3296
Fax: (715) 528-3341
(Florence County HS)
501 Lake Avenue
Post Office Box 170
Florence, WI 54121

FOND DU LAC COUNTY
(920) 929-3400
Fax: (920) 929-3447
Fond du Lac County SS
87 Vincent Street
Post Office Box 1196
Fond du Lac, WI 54936-1196

FOREST COUNTY
(715) 478-3351
Fax: (715) 478-2847
Forest County SS
Forest County Courthouse
200 East Madison Street
Crandon, WI 54520

GRANT COUNTY
(608) 723-2136
Fax: (608) 723-4834
Grant County SS
8820 Highway35 & 61 South
Post Office Box 447
Lancaster, WI 53813

GREEN COUNTY
(608) 328-9393
Fax: (608) 328-9480
Green County HS
Pleasant View Complex
N3152 State Road 81
Monroe, WI 53566

GREEN LAKE COUNTY
(920) 294-4070
Fax: (920) 294-4139
Green Lake County HHS
500 Lake Steel Street
Post Office Box 588
Green Lake, WI 54941-0588

IOWA COUNTY
(608) 935-9311
Fax: (608) 935-9754
Iowa County SS
109 West Fountain Street
Dodgeville, WI 53533

IRON COUNTY
(715) 561-3636
Fax: (715) 561-2128
Iron County HS
Courthouse
300 Taconite Street
Hurley, WI 54534

JACKSON COUNTY
(715) 284-4301
Fax: (715) 284-7713
Jackson County HS
420 HIGHWAY 54 West
Post Office Box 457
Black River Falls, WI 54615

JEFFERSON COUNTY
(920) 674-7500
Fax: (920) 674-7520
Workforce Development Center of Jefferson County
874 Collins Road
Jefferson, WI 53549

JUNEAU COUNTY
(608) 847-2400
Fax: (608) 847-9421
Juneau County HS
Courthouse Annex
220 East LaCrosse Street
Mauston, WI 53948

KENOSHA COUNTY
(262) 697-4500
Fax: (262) 697-4563
Kenosha County DCF
Kenosha County Job Center
8600 Sheridan Road
Post Office Box 4248
Kenosha, WI 53141-4248

KEWAUNEE COUNTY
(920) 388-3777
Fax: (920) 388-2122
Kewaunee County HS
510 Kilbourn Street
Kewaunee, WI 54216

LACROSSE COUNTY
(608) 785-6000
Fax: (608) 785-5565
LaCrosse County HS
300 North 4th Street
LaCrosse, WI 54602-4002

LAFAYETTE COUNTY
(608) 776-4900
Fax: (608) 776-4915
Lafayette County HS
Post Office Box 206
627 Main Street
Darlington, WI 53530

LANGLADE COUNTY
(715) 627-4750
Fax: (715) 627-6295
Langlade County SS
1225 Langlade Road
Antigo, WI 54409

LINCOLN COUNTY
(715) 536-6200
Fax: (715) 536-2753
Lincoln County SS
Post Office Box 547
Merrill, WI 54452

MANITOWOC COUNTY
(920) 683-4400
Fax: (920) 683-4908
Manitowoc County HS
926 South 8th Street
Post Office Box 1177
Manitowoc, WI 54221-1177

MARATHON COUNTY
(715) 261-7500
Fax: (715) 261-7510
Marathon County SS
400 East Thomas Street
Wausau, WI 54403-6498

MARINETTE COUNTY
(715) 732-7700
Fax: (715) 732-7766
Marinette County HS
2500 Hall Avenue, Suite B
Marinette, WI 54143

MARQUETTE COUNTY
(608) 297-7550
Fax: (608) 297-2148
Marquette County SS
PO Box 99
Montello, WI 53949

MENOMINEE COUNTY
(715) 799-3861
Fax: (715) 799-3517
Menominee County HS
Social Services Bldg.
Post Office Box 280
Keshena, WI 54135-0280

MILWAUKEE COUNTY
(414) 289-5700
Fax: (414) 289-5788
Milwaukee County HS
1220 Vliet Street
Milwaukee, WI 53205

MONROE COUNTY
(608) 269-8600
Fax: (608) 269-8935
Monroe County HS
Community Services Center, Bldg. A.
14301 CTH B, Box 19
Sparta, WI 54656-4509

OCONTO COUNTY
(920) 834-7000
Fax: (920) 834-6889
Oconto County HS
501 Park Avenue
Oconto, WI 54153-1612

ONEIDA COUNTY
(715) 362-5695
Fax: (715) 362-7910
Oneida County SS
Oneida County Courthouse
PO Box 400
Rhinelander, WI 54501

OUTAGAMIE COUNTY
(920) 832-5168
Fax: (920) 832-4779
Outagamie County HHS
401 South Elm Street
Appleton, WI 54911-5985

OZAUKEE COUNTY
(262) 238-8200 or 284-8200
Fax: (262) 238-8103 or 284-8103
Ozaukee County SS
Administration Center
121 West Main Street
Post Office Box 994
Port Washington, WI 53074-0994

PEPIN COUNTY
(715) 672-8941
Fax: (715) 672-8593
Pepin County HS
740 Seventh Avenue, West
Post Office Box 39
Durand, WI 54736-0039

PIERCE COUNTY
(715) 273-6788
Fax: (715) 273-6787
Pierce County HS
388 West Main Street
Post Office Box 670
Ellsworth, WI 54011

POLK COUNTY
(715) 485-8400
Fax: (715) 485-8490
Polk County SS
300 Polk Plaza, Suite 110
Balsam Lake, WI 54810

PORTAGE COUNTY
(715) 345-5350
Fax: (715) 345-5966
Portage County HHS
817 Whiting Avenue
Stevens Point, WI 54481

PRICE COUNTY
(715) 339-2158
Fax: (715) 339-4018
Price County CHS
104 South Eyder Avenue
PO Box 88
1045 Eyder Avenue
Phillips, WI 54555

RACINE COUNTY
(262) 638-6353
Fax: (262) 638-6376
Racine County HS
1717 Taylor Avenue
Racine, WI 53403-2497

RICHLAND COUNTY
(608) 647-8821
Fax: (608) 647-6611
Richland County SS
221 West Seminary Street
Post Office Box 673
Richland Center, WI 53581

ROCK COUNTY
(608) 741-3400
Fax: (608) 741-3429
Rock County HS
1900 Center Avenue
Janesville, WI 53546

RUSK COUNTY
(715) 532-2116
Fax: (715) 532-2126
Rusk County SS
311 East Miner Avenue, Suite C240
Ladysmith, WI 54848

ST CROIX COUNTY
(715) 246-8257
Fax: (715) 246-8220
St. Croix County HHS
1445 North 4th Street
New Richmond, WI 54017

SAUK COUNTY
(608) 355-4200
Fax: (608) 355-4299
Sauk County HS
505 Broadway
Post Office Box 29
Baraboo, WI 53913

SAWYER COUNTY
(715) 634-4806
Fax: (715) 634-5387
Sawyer County HS
105 East 4th Street
Post Office Box 730
Hayward, WI 54843

SHAWANA COUNTY
(715) 526-4700
Fax: (715) 524-2573
Shawano County SS
311 North Main Street,
Post Office Box 434
Shawano, WI 54166-0434

SHEBOYGAN COUNTY
(920) 459-6400
Fax: (920) 459-4353
Sheboygan County HHS
1011 North 8th Street
Sheboygan, WI 53081

TAYLOR COUNTY
(715) 748-3332
Fax: (715) 748-3342
Taylor County HS
540 East College Street
Medford, WI 54451-2027

TREMPEALEAU COUNTY
(715) 538-2311, ext. 290
Fax: (715) 538-4274
Trempealeau County SS
Post Office Box 67
Whitehall, WI 54773-0067

VERNON COUNTY
(608) 637-5210
Fax: (608) 637-5505
Vernon County DHS
Post Office Box 823
Viroqua, WI 54665-0823

VILAS COUNTY
(715) 479-3668
Fax: (715) 479-3728
Vilas County SSD
330 Court Street
Eagle River, WI 54521

WALWORTH COUNTY

(262) 741-3300
Fax: (262) 741-3320
Walworth County DHS
3955 Highway NN
Box 1006
Elkhorn, WI 53121-1006

WASHBURN COUNTY

(715) 468-4747
Fax: (715) 468-4753
Washburn County DSS
Post Office Box 250
Shell Lake, WI 54871

WASHINGTON COUNTY

(262) 335-4610
Fax: (262) 335-4709
Washington County SS
333 East Washington Street, Suite 3100
West Bend, WI 53095

WAUKESHA COUNTY

(262) 695-7945 Waukesha County HHS
500 Riverview Avenue
Waukesha, WI 53188

WAUPACA COUNTY

(715) 258-6300
Fax: (715) 258-6409
Waupaca County HHS
811 Harding Street
Waupaca, WI 54981-2080

WAUSHARA COUNTY
(920) 787-3303
Fax: (920) 787-0421
Waushara County SS
230 West Park Street
Post Office Box 898
Wautoma, WI 54982

WINNEBAGO COUNTY
(920) 236-4600
Fax: (920) 236-1222
Winnebago County SS
220 Washington Avenue
Box 2646
Oshkosh, WI 54903-2646

WOOD COUNTY
(715) 421-8600
Fax: (715) 421-8693
(715) 387-6374
Fax: (715) 387-6672
Wood County SS
Courthouse, 400 Market Street
Post Office Box 8095
Wisconsin Rapids, WI 54495-8095
-AND-
630 South Central Avenue, Suite 404
Marshfield, WI 54449

WYOMING DEPARTMENT OF FAMILY SERVICES
COUNTY/REGION FIELD OFFICES

ALBANY
Laramie Plains Civic Center
710 Garfield Street, Suite 220
Laramie, WY 82070
(307) 745-7324
Fax: (307) 742-8848

BIG HORN
616 Second Avenue North
Greybull, WY 82426
(307) 765-9453
Fax: (307) 765-2330

CAMPBELL
1901 Energy Court
Gillette, WY 82716
(307) 682-7277
Fax: (307) 687-1889

CARBON
Carbon Building
Third and Buffalo
Box 2409
Rawlins, WY 82301
(307) 328-0612
Fax: (307) 328-2801

CONVERSE
530 Oak Street
Douglas, WY 82301
(307) 358-3138
Fax: (307) 358-4238

CONVERSE
925 West Birch Box 26
Glenrock, WY 82637
(307) 436-9068

CROOK
102 North Fifth Box 57
Sundance, WY 82729
(307) 283-2014
Fax: (307) 283-1606

FREMONT
201 North 4th Street
Lander, WY 82520
(307) 332-4038
Fax: (307) 332-4806

FREMONT
120 North 6th Street, East
Riverton, WY 82501
(307) 856-6521
Fax: (307) 856-7937

GOSHEN
1618 East M Street
Torrington, WY 82240
(307) 532-2191
Fax: (307) 532-4666

HOT SPRINGS
403 Big Horn
Thermopolis, WY 82443
(307) 864-2158
Fax: (307) 864-2651

JOHNSON
381 North Main Street Box J
Buffalo, WY 82443
(307) 684-5513
Fax: (307) 684-7966

LARAMIE
1710 Capitol Avenue
Cheyenne, WY 82002
(307) 777-7921
Fax: (307) 777-5190

LINCOLN (SOUTH)
1100 Pine Avenue, Box 470
Kemmerer, WY 83101
(307) 877-6670
Fax: (307) 877-4332

LINCOLN (NORTH)
631 Washington
PO Box 1336
Afton, WY 83110
(307) 886-9232
Fax: (307) 886-3101

NATRONA
851 Werner Court, Suite 200
Casper, WY 82601
(307) 473-3900
Fax: (307) 473-3967

NIOBRARA
905 South Main, Box 389
Lusk, WY 82225
(307) 334-2153
*note, this is a temporary address

PARK
1301 Rumsey Street
Cody, WY 82414
(307) 587-6246
Fax: (307) 527-7183

PARK
109 West 14th Street
Powell, WY 82435
(307) 754-2245
Fax: (307) 754-9439

PLATTE
975 Gilchrist Street
Wheatland, WY 82201
(307) 322-3790
Fax: (307) 322-4125

SHERIDAN
16 West 8th Street
Box 785
Sheridan, WY 82801
(307) 672-2404
Fax: (307) 672-8948

SUBLETTE
111 North Sublette, Box 1070
Pinedale, WY 82941
(307) 367-4124
Fax: (307) 367-6774

SWEETWATER
1682 Sunset Drive
Rock Springs, WY 82901
(307) 362-5630 and (307) 382-5916
Fax: (307) 382-5917

TETON
145 West Gill, Box 547
Jackson, WY 83001
(307) 733-7757
Fax: (307) 733-0082

UINTA
350 City View Drive, Suite 206
Evanston, WY 82930
(307) 789-2756
Fax: (307) 789-2165

UINTA
111 West Owens Street, Box 848
Lyman, WY 82937
(307) 786-4011
Fax: (307) 787-6359

WASHAKIE
1700 Robertson
Worland, WY 82401
(307) 347-6181
Fax: (307) 347-6184

WESTON
1517 West Main
Newcastle, WY 82701
(307) 746-4657
Fax: (307) 746-2588

Glossary

Annuity-A contract between an insurance company and an individual in which an insurer agrees, for a price, to make regular payments to an individual for a fixed time period or for life.

Asset-an item of cash value, which is owned.

Assignment-the transfer of title, interests or proceeds from the applicant/recipient to the Department of Social Services.

Available Net Income-gross income less standard allowable Medicaid deductions.

Available Resource-liquid or an easily liquidable resource, which is considered as part of the total resource allowance.

Budgeting-process which a Medicaid Representative uses to evaluate a client's income and resources to determine Medicaid eligibility.

Burial Fund/Burial Arrangements-revocable burial contracts, burial trusts, other burial arrangements, cash accounts, or other financial instruments (documents which have a definite cash value) clearly designated for burial expenses.

Burial Space-conventional grave sites, crypts, mausoleums, urns, vaults, caskets and other repositories, which are customarily and traditionally used for the remains of deceased persons.

Cash Value of Life Insurance-amount that the insurer will pay upon cancellation of the policy before death or maturity. This value usually increases with the age of the policy.

Citizenship-Medicaid may only be authorized for individuals who were born in this country, naturalized as citizens, are legal aliens who are permanently residing in the United States under the color of the law, or are legal aliens admitted for permanent residence.

Clearance Report-report which matches information about each individual applying for assistance taken from the applications. The resulting computer printout is a report listing the names and identifying data of any individual who appears to be the same or very similar to the applicant according to such statistics as name date of birth, social security number. The clearance report is obtained through the process of Application Registry.

Client Identification Number-client specific system generated number permanently assigned to each individual who has ever applied.

Community Spouse-legally married person who is not living in a medical institution or nursing facility, and has a spouse residing in a medical institution or medical facility.

Community Spouse Resource Allowance-amount of a couples' total joint resources, which is attributed to the community spouse at the time that Medicaid eligibility is determined for the institutionalized spouse.

Community Spouse Monthly Income Allowance-the minimum monthly income allowance is the amount of income that may be attributed to the community spouse each month to bring him/her up to the income level.

Community Based Waivered Services-(**Nursing Home Without Walls**) Home care services for individuals who are ill or disabled and remain at home as long as possible.

Conservator-manages only the financial resources of an incapacitated individual.

Continuous Period of Institutionalization-at least 30 consecutive days of institutionalization in a qualified medical institution and/or nursing facility.

Co-Payment-third party insurance provision, by which both the insured and the insurer share the medical expenses.

Contribution to Cost of Care-net amount of income paid to the medical facility each month for applicant's share of the cost.

Contiguous Property-land, which is adjoining the homestead of an applicant and can be separately liquidated.

Custodial care–care for the purpose of meeting personal needs and could be provided by persons without professional skills or training. May include help in walking, getting in and out of bed, and bathing, dressing, eating, and taking medicine.

Dependent Family Member-a minor child, dependent adult child, dependent parent, or dependent sibling of either spouse, who is living with the community spouse and who is listed on the federal tax form as a dependent (IRS tax dependent) of the community spouse.

Earned Income-income, which is received as a result of work activity.

Excess Resources/Assets-resources owned and available that are over the allowable standards.

Excess Income-(Spend down) Income that is above the allowable standard and applied to the cost of care.

Face Value Life Insurance-the basic death benefit or maturity amount, which is specified on the face of the policy.

Fair Hearing-a formal administrative hearing by which the applicant may dispute a decision made by the Medicaid department.

Fair Market Value-of property (real and personal) is the amount for which the property can be expected to sell on the open market in the geographic area involved and under existing economic conditions at the time of the determination.

Family Member Allowance-the amount of income an institutionalized individual can give to a dependent family member other than a community spouse.

Federal Poverty Level-annual Federal Poverty Levels (FPL) computed by the Office of Management and Budget published in the Federal Register.

Financial Assessment-an assessment of all assets as of the date of admission to the nursing home. This is available from the Medicaid department upon request.

First of the Month Rule-point in time at which to value a resource.

Guardian-is appointed to make personal care decisions for the incapacitated individual.

Homestead-home owned and occupied by the applicant and his/her spouse as a principal residence.

Immediate Family-an individual's minor and adult children, stepchildren, adopted children, brothers, sisters, parents, adoptive parents and the spouse of those individuals.

Power of Attorney-a document by which one person gives legal authority to another to act as an agent on their behalf.

Lien-a hold or claim upon property of another as a security form some debt or charge.

Life Estate-a life estate conveys to an individual or individuals certain rights to property, which expire upon the death of the owner or of another person.

Life Insurance-contract between the owner of a policy and an insurance company, whereby the company agrees, in return for periodic premium payments, to pay a specified sum to the designated beneficiary upon the death of the insured.

Look Back Period-the 36 months of financial records prior to the date nursing home coverage is needed. The look-back period for a Trust is 60 months.

Medicaid-is a State and Federal program that will pay most nursing home costs for people with limited income and assets Medicaid will only pay for nursing home care provided in Medicaid certified facilities.

Medicare-is a Federal health insurance program through the Social Security Office for those individuals 65 or older, and those disabled for at least two years.

Medical Assessment-an assessment to determine the level of care needed.

Mineral Rights-is an ownership interest in certain natural resources, which are usually obtained from the ground such as coal, sulfur, petroleum, sand, natural gas, etc.

Miller Trusts-income trusts designed for individuals who otherwise would be over the income level in income-capped states.

Nursing Home Escrow Accounts-an amount deposited in an interest bearing account at the nursing home for those individuals who are self-pay.

Nursing Home-a residence certified to provide different levels of care to meet the needs of acutely or chronically ill individuals.

Ombudsman-an impartial fact-finder whose job is to assure that individuals receive fair treatment while residing in a nursing home and other long term facilities.

Permanent Absence-someone who is in a medical institution and a medical determination has been made that the person is not expected to return home.

Personal Needs Allowance-a specified amount of money set aside each month from income, for the individual in the nursing home to use for personal needs. This specified amount varies from state to state.

Power of Attorney-a power of attorney is a document by which one person gives legal authority to another to act as an agent on their behalf.

Prepaid Burial Contract-is an agreement in which an individual prepays his/her burial expenses.

Rebuttal-written statement that documents a desire to rebut the presumption of ownership interest or transfer.

Recertification/Reapplication-investigation and documentation at intervals by which continuing eligibility for Medicaid is established. Individual states determine the frequency.

Resource-cash or liquid assets and real or personal property.

Snapshot Rule-a determination of a couple's resources on the first day of continuous institutionalization or from the time of the Medicaid application, whichever comes first.

Savings Bond-backed by the federal government. There are several series E, I, J, H, which normally can be quickly converted to cash.

Spend down-income or resources per month above the established Medicaid standards. This amount is applied to the cost of care.

Stock-a negotiable instrument, which represents ownership in a corporation. The value of the stock varies frequently.

Temporary Absence-a period of time when a person is institutionalized but expected to return home. A person is presumed to be temporarily absent when placed in an acute care hospital.

Telephone Screening-call to the Medicaid Representative to discuss applying for Medicaid.

Third Party Insurance-contract or agreement by an individual, institution, corporation, public or private agency who may be liable to pay all or part of the cost of medical services provided to the insured.

Timber Rights-permit an individual to cut and remove freestanding trees from property owned by another.

Transfer of Resources-giving away or selling resources for less than fair market value. Presumed by Medicaid to be for the sole purpose of becoming eligible for Medicaid.

Transfer Penalty-period of ineligibility based on the transfer of assets.

Trust-is property, real or personal, held by one party for the benefit of another.

Unearned Income-income, which is paid because of a legal or moral obligation such as pensions, benefits, interest and other types of payments.

Verification-the process of proving an applicant's situation as stated by the applicant.

Waivered Services-services provided in the home which otherwise would require institutional care.

Index

6% Rate of Return, 31, 35

Acute Care, 2, 30, 691

Aid and Attendance, 42

Annuity, 27

Application, 1, 3-5, 8-9, 11-18, 20, 24-25, 28, 46, 48, 51, 55-56, 358, 367, 686, 690

Asset, 12, 23-24, 30-32, 34

Assignment, 685

Available Net Income, 685

Available Resource, 685

Bank Records, 19, 51

Book Value, 27

Budgeting, 685

Burial Arrangements, 685

Burial Fund, 685

Burial Space, 26

Business Income, 41-42, 44

Cash Deposit, 4

Cash Value of Life Insurance, 686

Citizenship, 686

Clearance Report, 686

Client Identification Number, 686

Community Based Waivered Services, 1, 3, 5, 11, 686

Community Spouse, 23-25, 38-39, 47, 686-688

Community Spouse Monthly Income Allowance, 686

Community Spouse Resource Allowance, 686

Conservator, 687

Contiguous Property, 687

Continuous Period of Institutionalization, 687

Contribution to Cost of Care, 687

Co-Payment, 687

Court Order, 25

Custodial Care, 2, 687

Deeds, 19, 47, 51

Department of Human Services, 4, 61, 65, 68, 95, 175, 199, 215, 399, 419, 480, 495, 523, 601, 617, 631

Dependent Family Member, 687, 688

Documentation, 17-18, 20, 22, 30-31, 34, 40-41, 44, 51, 690

Earned Income, 687

Equity Value, 31-32

Escrow Account, 28

Excess Assets687

Excess Income, 687

Excess Resources, 687

Excluded Asset, 687

Face Value of Life Insurance, 687

Face-to-Face Interview, 8, 17-18, 22

Fair Hearing, 21-22, 25, 34, 47, 55

Fair Market Value, 20, 30, 32, 34

Family Member Allowance, 688

Federal Poverty Level, 688

Financial Assessment, 688

Financial Records, 9, 19-20, 26-27, 30, 51, 689

First of the Month Rule, 24, 35

Generic Application, 11

Going Nursing Home Rate, 32

Group Insurance, 29

Guardian, 19, 38

Home Maintenance Allowance, 38
Homestead, 24, 30, 687
Household Goods, 28
Immediate Family, 688
Income, 2, 4, 8, 12-14, 16, 18-21, 23, 25, 27, 29-34, 37-47, 49, 51, 53,
          56, 289, 302, 685-690
Income Cap State, 44
Income Producing Property, 31
Income Trusts, 38
Inheritance, 29, 47
Initial Phone Screening, 29
Interest Income, 25, 40, 46
Interview, 7-8, 15, 17-18, 22, 30, 358
Inventory*****
Irrevocable, 24, 28, 38
Lien, 688
Life Estate, 34-35, 689
Life Expectancy Chart, 27
Life Insurance, 19, 24, 26, 29, 43, 46-47, 51
Liquid Resource, 23
Look Back Period, 26, 34-35
Lump Sum, 14, 29, 40, 47
Married Couple, 25, 35
Maximum Income Payment, 43
Maximum Resource Level, 24-25
Medicaid Regulations, 31, 43
Medical Assessment, 3, 5
Medicare, 2, 4-5, 8-9, 13-14, 19, 37, 51, 56
Medicare Cut Letter, 9
Miller Trusts, 38
Mineral Rights, 26
Mortgage Income, 43

Move, 48-49

Net Worth, 7

Non-Liquid Resource, 23

Nursing Home, 1-5, 7-9, 11, 20-21, 23-26, 28-29, 32-35, 37-39, 42,
        45-48, 174-176, 197, 353, 365-366, 472, 686, 688-690

Nursing Home Escrow Accounts, 689

Nursing Home Without Walls, 3, 175-176, 686

Office for the Aging, 4, 20, 64, 79

Ombudsman, 71-73, 75-77, 80

Ombudsmen, 4, 71

Outstanding Medical Bills, 8

Permanent Absence, 690

Personal Effects, 28

Personal Needs Allowance, 37, 42

Personal Needs Deduction, 37

Phone Screening, 7-8, 10, 29

Power of Attorney, 19, 51, 690

Pre-admission Screening, 3

Premeditated Transfer, 34

Prepaid Burial Contract, 690

Real Estate, 8, 13, 19, 26, 30, 32, 35, 51

Reapplication, 46, 49, 53

Rebuttal, 21, 34

Recertification, 46-47, 49, 53, 690

Redetermination, 46, 49

Rental Property Income, 41, 44

Residency Requirements, 11, 16

Resource, 4, 12, 16, 23-25, 27-32, 34-35, 43, 47, 53, 500, 685-686, 688

Retirement Pensions, 19, 40, 43

Revocable, 27-28

Risk, 25

Safe Deposit Box, 20

Savings Bond, 690
Schedule A, 30
Self-Employment Income, 46
Settlement, 29, 47
Shelter Allowance, 19, 39
Snapshot Rule, 690
Social Security, 2, 12, 14, 18-19, 37, 40, 43, 45, 51, 53, 56, 686, 689
Spend down, 24, 687
Spousal Impoverishment Law, 23
State Allowance, 8
Statements of Responsibility, 14
Stock, 24, 691
Telephone Screening, 691
Temporary Absence, 691
Term Insurance, 29
Third Party Insurance, 687, 691
Timber Rights, 691
Trade-in Value, 27
Transfer of Resources, 8, 27, 32, 35
Transfer Penalty, 691
Trust, 8, 13, 26-27, 30-31, 33, 38, 40, 51, 689
Trust Assets, 30
Unearned Income, 691
Unisex Life Estate and Remainder Interest Tables, 34
Vehicles, 20, 26-27, 51
Verification, 19-20, 29, 31, 41, 45-47, 51
Veteran's Benefits, 42-43
Waivered Services, 1, 3, 5, 11, 14, 26, 686
Windfall, 14, 29, 47

www.ingramcontent.com/pod-product-compliance
Lightning Source LLC
Chambersburg PA
CBHW020717180526

45163CB00001B/11